Everything You Need to Know to Manage Type 2 Diabetes

Other Titles in the New Glucose Revolution Series

For the definitive overview of the glycemic index . . .
- *The Low GI Handbook: The New Glucose Revolution Guide to the Long-term Health Benefits of Low GI Eating*

For a focus on recipes, shopping and the GI in the larger nutrition picture . . .
- *The New Glucose Revolution Low GI Vegetarian Cookbook*
- *The New Glucose Revolution Low GI Family Cookbook*
- *The New Glucose Revolution Life Plan*
- *The New Glucose Revolution Low GI Guide to Sugar and Energy*

For a basic introduction to the GI, plus the top 100 low GI foods . . .
- *The New Glucose Revolution Low GI Eating Made Easy: The Beginner's Guide to Eating with the Glycemic Index*

For a focus on weight loss . . .
- *The Low GI Diet Revolution: The Definitive Science-Based Weight Loss Plan*
- *The Low GI Diet Cookbook: 100 Simple, Delicious Smart-Carb Recipes— The Proven Way to Lose Weight and Eat for Lifelong Health*
- *The New Glucose Revolution Low GI Guide to Losing Weight*

For a focus on the GI and specific health conditions . . .
- *The New Glucose Revolution Low GI Gluten-Free Eating Made Easy: The Essential Guide to the Glycemic Index and Gluten-Free Living*
- *The New Glucose Revolution Low GI Guide to the Metabolic Syndrome and Your Heart: The Only Authoritative Guide to Using the Glycemic Index for Better Heart Health*
- *The New Glucose Revolution What Makes My Blood Glucose Go Up . . . and Down?: 101 Frequently Asked Questions about Your Blood Glucose Level*
- *The Low GI Guide to Living Well with PCOS*

Everything You Need to Know to Manage

Type 2 Diabetes

SIMPLE STEPS *for* **SURVIVING** *and* **THRIVING** *with the* **LOW GI PLAN**

JENNIE BRAND-MILLER
KAYE FOSTER-POWELL
STEPHEN COLAGIURI
ALAN BARCLAY

Da Capo

LIFE
LONG

A Member of the Perseus Books Group

Copyright © 2007, 2015 by Jennie Brand-Miller, Kaye Foster-Powell, Stephen Colagiuri, Alan Barclay

Original text design by Pindar NZ

Cataloging-in-Publication data for this book is available from the Library of Congress.

This is a completely revised edition of *The New Glucose Revolution for Diabetes*, published in 2007 by Da Capo Press. This edition was first published in Australia and New Zealand as *Low GI Diet: Managing Type 2 Diabetes* and is published in the United States by arrangement with Hachette Australia.

ISBN: 978-0-7382-1847-2 (paperback)
ISBN: 978-0-7382-1848-9 (e-book)

Published by Da Capo Press
A Member of the Perseus Books Group
www.dacapopress.com

Note: The information in this book is true and complete to the best of our knowledge. This book is intended only as an informative guide for those wishing to know more about health issues. In no way is this book intended to replace, countermand, or conflict with the advice given to you by your own physician. The ultimate decision concerning care should be made between you and your doctor. We strongly recommend you follow his or her advice. Information in this book is general and is offered with no guarantees on the part of the authors or Da Capo Press. The authors and publisher disclaim all liability in connection with the use of this book.

Da Capo Press books are available at special discounts for bulk purchases in the U.S. by corporations, institutions, and other organizations. For more information, please contact the Special Markets Department at the Perseus Books Group, 2300 Chestnut Street, Suite 200, Philadelphia, PA, 19103, or call (800) 810-4145, ext. 5000, or e-mail special.markets@perseusbooks.com.

10 9 8 7 6 5 4 3 2 1

Contents

Introduction

Diabetes has been around for thousands of years and was once relatively rare. Its literal meaning is "to pass through"—referring to the passing of liquids through the body. The ancient Egyptians recommended that those suffering from "the passing of too much urine" eat a diet of fruit, grain and sweet beer. The Greeks, who mistakenly thought it was a weakness of the kidneys, prescribed exercise, "preferably on horseback."

Diabetes is no longer rare. In fact it is one of the fastest growing diseases in the world. About 382 million people in the world have diabetes, and that number is expected to almost double in the next 20 years. It can cause heart disease, blindness and kidney failure, and it can lead to amputation. It can be a killer.

In the US currently, at least 1 out of 3 people will develop type 2 diabetes in their lifetime. Every day more than 4,500 people, including children, are being diagnosed with diabetes. Shockingly, 9 out of 10 people with prediabetes don't know they have it. Millions of dollars are being spent by governments in treating, managing and preventing the epidemic, but the way to stem the tide really begins with us as individuals.

In this day and age we all have immense potential for good health, but many people are uninformed or confused by what's involved in a healthy lifestyle. Living well with diabetes doesn't mean being on a "diet." It means eating nutritious foods—and not eating whatever happens to be in front of you. It means making smarter food choices. And it means making the effort to move more.

In the last decade research has yielded overwhelming evidence that lifestyle changes such as eating well and increasing physical activity can make a real difference to our risk of developing type 2 diabetes and to the quality of our health if we already have it. It's never too late to make a difference. There is the potential to turn back the clock.

How to use this book

There are many types of diabetes and many different approaches to managing it. This book is a diet and lifestyle guide to living well with diabetes or prediabetes, and there are many ways to do this. Our aim is to translate the current scientific evidence about managing and preventing diabetes into an accessible, practical resource, giving you the information you can use to discover what works best for you.

The book sets out clearly and simply what you need to eat and do to:

- Reduce your risk of developing diabetes
- Improve your cardiovascular health
- Keep your blood glucose levels, blood pressure and blood fats under control, and
- Maintain a healthy body.

Part 1: So your doctor has told you that you have diabetes or prediabetes spells out the differences between the various types of diabetes, tells you how they are diagnosed and explains key aspects of their management.

Part 2: What *you* can do to take control of the things in your life you can change describes the five fundamental steps to take to maintain a healthy lifestyle.

Part 3: Living with diabetes, prediabetes and the metabolic syndrome consists of sections on each type of diabetes and includes daily food guides, sample menu plans and the answers to frequently asked questions.

Diabetes is a complex condition and there are aspects of its management—such as blood glucose monitoring, medications and insulin—which are not covered in detail. Nor do we cover management of diabetes complications (we hope this book will mean you never get them). The information in this handbook is not intended to take the place of individual consultation with your doctor or diabetes health professionals.

We hope that this book will help you to manage your diabetes successfully or turn back the clock with prediabetes. We wish you every success in preventing or managing diabetes.

Alan Barclay
Jennie Brand-Miller
Stephen Colagiuri
Kaye Foster-Powell

PART 1:

So your doctor has told you that you have diabetes or prediabetes

Chapter 1
What you need to know about type 2 diabetes

Type 2 diabetes is a chronic condition. In simple terms, it means that your blood glucose (sometimes you will hear it called blood sugar, but it is the same thing) is too high. You can manage your diabetes successfully, but it will never go away and as yet there's no cure.

The most important thing to keep in mind is that having diabetes need not stop you from enjoying life to the full. However, it is important that you:

- Are informed about your body and blood glucose levels (BGLs), and
- Take control of the things in your life you can change (like what you eat, how active you are and quitting smoking).

Understanding what diabetes does to your body and knowing what you need to do to manage it will allow you to live well and reduce your risk of complications. And that's what this book is about. In Part 2 we give you the five key steps to managing your diabetes successfully, and in Part 3 we get down to exactly what to eat for better blood glucose with meal plans and food guides for adults, children and pregnant women.

What you need to know about your body and blood glucose levels

Your diet is a key factor in managing diabetes successfully. Here's why.

Our bodies run on fuel, just like a car runs on gas. In fact, our bodies burn a special mix of fuels that come from the protein, fat and carbohydrate in the foods we eat.

When we eat carbohydrate-rich foods such as bread, potatoes and other starchy vegetables, pasta, rice and other grains, noodles, breakfast cereals and fruit, our body converts them into a sugar called glucose during digestion. This glucose is then absorbed from our intestine and becomes the fuel that circulates in our bloodstream, and that's when our blood glucose levels rise. At this point, our pancreas gets the message to release a hormone called insulin to drive glucose out of the bloodstream and into our body's cells where our body can either use it as an immediate source of energy or convert it into glycogen (the name for the storage form of glucose) or into fat.

Glucose matters

Glucose is a universal fuel for our body cells, the primary fuel source for our brain, red blood cells and a growing fetus, and the main source of energy during strenuous exercise. We can't live without it.

Sometimes glucose levels build up in the bloodstream and lead to high blood glucose levels and a diagnosis of diabetes or prediabetes. There are two reasons for this.

- When the insulin can't do its job properly, it is called **insulin resistance**.

- When the pancreas does not produce enough insulin to reduce blood glucose levels, it is called **insulin deficiency**.

Insulin resistance, which occurs without you even knowing it, is thought to be a contributing factor in the development of diabetes. Having insulin resistance means that your muscle and liver cells are not good at taking up glucose from the blood, unless there's a truckload of insulin about. This makes the beta cells in your pancreas work overtime to produce extra insulin so that your muscle cells get enough glucose for making energy. Once your beta cells are unable to produce enough insulin to overcome the resistance, you get high blood glucose levels . . . and along with that, the diagnosis of diabetes. In Chapter 2 we look at insulin resistance in more detail and explain how it is diagnosed.

Many factors are being identified as contributing to this failure of the beta cells, and it is believed to be at least partly in your genes. This is why diabetes is more common among certain groups. African-Americans, Hispanic Americans, Native Americans, Aboriginal Australians or Torres Strait Islanders, Maoris, Pacific Islanders, Southeast Asians and Asian Indians are at a greater risk than people from an Anglo-Celtic background.

Two other key risk factors for diabetes are:

- Your age. Older people are more at risk than younger people.
- Your lifestyle. Being overweight and not exercising enough can contribute to the development of type 2 diabetes, especially in families where someone already has diabetes. In fact, about 80 percent of people with type 2 diabetes are overweight.

Occasionally there are other causes of diabetes. There are some medical disorders that cause secondary diabetes, such as pancreatitis (inflammation of the pancreas) and acromegaly (due to excessive production of growth hormone).

A number of medications also increase the risk of diabetes—the most important of these are the glucocorticoids or "steroids" that are often used by people with severe asthma or arthritis. People who need to take certain antipsychotic drugs for mental disorders or anti-HIV drugs for AIDS may also increase their risk of developing type 2 diabetes.

Did you know?

The risk of dying from a heart attack is increased 2–3 times if you have diabetes.

Diagnosing diabetes

The main symptoms of diabetes are:

- Increased thirst
- Tiredness
- Blurred vision
- Leg cramps
- Increased urine output
- Always feeling hungry
- Itching, skin infections, cuts that won't heal, and
- Unexplained weight loss (which may occur when glucose levels are very high).

However, most people with type 2 diabetes, especially early on, *have no obvious symptoms at all.*

Diabetes is diagnosed by a blood test. Diagnosing and treating diabetes early is an important way to prevent complications. If your doctor suspects diabetes, either because of your symptoms or because you are in one of the high risk groups, he or she will arrange for you to have a blood glucose test to measure your blood glucose level. This is best done after fasting overnight (no food between dinner and the test that is carried out the following morning).

- If the result of your test is very high and you have some of the symptoms we listed, that is all that your doctor needs to make the diagnosis.
- If the result of your test is moderately high, the test should be repeated to make sure of the diagnosis.
- If the result is a little bit higher than normal, you will need to have an oral glucose tolerance test to make the diagnosis. This involves fasting overnight, having a blood test to measure the fasting blood glucose, drinking a sweet drink of 75 grams of glucose and then measuring the blood glucose again 2 hours later.

Are you at risk of having undiagnosed diabetes?

For every 4 people with diabetes another 3 people are at high risk of developing diabetes. Having diabetes and not knowing about it is a serious risk to your health. About 1 in 4 people already have signs of permanent damage from diabetes by the time it is diagnosed. This is because they have had diabetes for a long time without knowing it, and their high blood glucose levels have been quietly causing problems.

If you can say yes to any of the following questions, you should be having annual checks of your blood glucose levels. This is the only way to find out if you have undiagnosed diabetes. Your doctor can arrange this.

- Are you over 45 years of age and have high blood pressure or high blood fats (cholesterol and/or triglycerides)?
- Are you over 40 years of age and overweight?
- Are you over 40 years of age and one or more members of the family has/had diabetes? (People with a family history of diabetes have 2 to 6 times the risk of developing type 2.)

- Are you over 55 years of age?
- Do you have heart disease or have you had a heart attack?
- Do you/have you had high blood glucose levels during pregnancy (Gestational Diabetes)?
- Do you have prediabetes: Impaired Fasting Glucose (IFG) or Impaired Glucose Tolerance (IGT)?
- Do you have Polycystic Ovarian Syndrome (PCOS)?
- Is your family background African-American, Hispanic/Latino, Native American, Asian American or Pacific Islander? The prevalence of type 2 diabetes is 2 to 6 times greater in these populations compared to people from a Caucasian background.
- Are you over 35 years of age and from the Pacific Islands, Indian subcontinent or have a Chinese background? (People born in certain overseas countries have a higher prevalence of diabetes.)

**Depression can be a significant problem
for people with diabetes**

Coming to terms with the changes that you have to make to accommodate diabetes has an impact. You may have times when you feel pretty distressed and unhappy with your lot. Making the transition from the "old before-diabetes self" to a "new managing-diabetes self" is difficult. Diabetes support groups, where you can talk to people who understand what you are going through, can really help you deal with low-level depression and anxiety. It's part of taking an active role in managing your diabetes, and this in itself can also be an antidote for depression.

However, some people are not able to overcome depression. If this is the case for you, seek help from a suitably qualified and experienced psychologist or psychiatrist.

Depression isn't just a fleeting feeling of sadness; it's a pervasive and relentless sense of despair. It is serious and you need to ask for help. Common symptoms of depression include:

- A general lack of interest in life
- Marked changes in your sleeping patterns, including having trouble sleeping
- Ongoing fatigue and listlessness
- Changes in your appetite: either a loss of appetite or over-eating
- Uncontrollable feelings of sadness, guilt, worthlessness or purposelessness
- An inability to concentrate on anything for longer than a few moments
- Suicidal thoughts, and
- Problems with sexual function (independent of any diabetes complications).

Talk to your doctor about getting professional help.

Chapter 2
What you need to know about insulin resistance

Insulin resistance means that your body does not react in a normal way to insulin in the blood—it is insensitive, or "partially deaf," to insulin. Just as we may shout to make a deaf person hear, the body makes more insulin in an effort to make it work. So moving glucose into cells requires more insulin. This is why high insulin levels are part and parcel of insulin resistance, which in turn can lead to high blood pressure, due to the effect of the high insulin levels on your kidneys.

While some insulin resistance is determined by your genes, what you do to your body is also very important. People who are overweight and do not exercise can often become insulin resistant.

How do you know if you have insulin resistance?

You probably have insulin resistance if you have two or more of the following:
- High waist circumference
- High blood pressure

- Low HDL (good) cholesterol levels
- Prediabetes
- High triglycerides, and
- High uric acid levels in your blood.

You might be normal weight but with a high waist circumference (more than 32 inches in women, more than 37 inches in men). This indicates excessive fat around the abdomen, which is also a heart health risk.

But the red flag is if your blood glucose and insulin levels are high.

Why is insulin resistance so common?

The answer is that both genes and environment play a role. People of Asian and African-American origin, and descendants of the original inhabitants of Australia and North and South America, appear to be more insulin resistant than those of Caucasian extraction, even when they are still young and lean. But regardless of ethnic background, insulin resistance develops as we age, probably because as we grow older we gain fat, become less active and lose some of our muscle mass.

What we eat plays an important role, too. Specifically, eating too much of the wrong kind of fat (saturated fat) and too much of the wrong kind of carbohydrate can increase your insulin resistance. If your carbohydrate intake is high, eating high GI foods can make pre-existing insulin resistance worse. In Chapter 10 we explain all about the GI (glycemic index).

Why is it a big deal?

The higher your insulin levels, the more carbohydrate you burn at the expense of fat. This is because insulin has two powerful actions: one is to "open the gates" so that glucose can flood into the cells and be used as the source of energy; the other is to *stop* the release of fat from fat stores. The burning of glucose reduces the burning of fat, and vice versa.

These two things keep going on even if you have insulin resistance because your body overcomes the extra hurdle by just pumping out more insulin into the blood. Unfortunately, the level that finally drives glucose into the cells is 2 to 10 times more than is needed to switch off the use of fat as a source of fuel.

If insulin levels are high all day long, as they are in insulin resistant and overweight people, the cells are constantly forced to use glucose as their fuel source. They draw it from either the blood or stored glycogen. The blood glucose level then swings from low to high and back again, playing havoc with appetite and triggering the release of stress hormones. And stores of carbohydrate in the liver and muscles also undergo major fluctuations over the course of the day.

When you don't get much chance to use fat as a source of fuel, it is not surprising that fat stores accumulate wherever they can:

- Inside the muscle cells (a sign of insulin resistance if you are not an elite athlete)
- In the blood (this means you have high triglycerides, and many people with diabetes or the metabolic syndrome have this)
- In the liver (non-alcoholic fatty liver), and
- Around the waist.

Insulin resistance gradually lays the foundations for heart attack and stroke.

Chapter 3
What you need to know about prediabetes

If you have prediabetes (the term used to describe impaired glucose tolerance and/or impaired fasting glucose), it means that you have blood glucose levels somewhere between normal and diabetes. It's diagnosed by either a fasting blood glucose test, a glucose tolerance test or a hemoglobin A1c test.

What does it mean?

- **Impaired fasting glucose** is a condition in which the fasting blood glucose level is elevated (between 100 and 126 mg/dL) after an overnight fast but is not high enough to be classified as diabetes.
- **Impaired glucose tolerance** is a condition in which the blood glucose level is elevated (greater than 140 mg/dL) 2 hours after an oral glucose tolerance test but is not high enough to be classified as diabetes (between 100 and 126 mg/dL).
- Prediabetes can also be diagnosed by a hemoglobin A1c test result of 5.7 to 6.4 percent (38.8 to 46.4 mmol/mol).

Left untreated, prediabetes can develop into type 2 diabetes. It also puts you at risk of some of the complications associated with diabetes, such as heart attacks and stroke.

The good news is that you can prevent, or at the very least delay, getting type 2 diabetes—and all of its complications. In fact we now know that 3 out of 5 people with prediabetes can prevent the development of type 2 diabetes by making some lifestyle changes such as losing weight, eating a healthy low GI diet, being more active and quitting smoking.

Be well; know your BGL (blood glucose level)

Normal ranges for:

Fasting glucose	60–100 mg/dL
Random glucose	<200 mg/dL
Two hours after 75g glucose load	<140 mg/dL
Glycated hemoglobin	<5.7 percent (38.8 mmol/mol)

Risk factors for developing prediabetes

If there's type 2 diabetes in your family, you probably already know that you have an increased chance of getting it too. But genes alone don't account for the current diabetes/prediabetes epidemic. Instead, it's the food we eat and our sedentary lifestyle. The most obvious trigger is that we're all getting heavier; and carrying extra body fat goes hand in hand with prediabetes and diabetes. People who are overweight, particularly around their middle, have up to three times more chance of developing diabetes than people who are in the healthy weight range.

Risk factors for prediabetes you cannot change

- A family history of diabetes
- Your ethnic background (people of African-American, Hispanic/Latino, Native American, Asian American and Pacific Island background have a greater risk)

- Having polycystic ovarian syndrome (PCOS)
- Having diabetes in pregnancy or giving birth to a big baby (more than 9 lbs)
- Having heart disease, angina, or having had a heart attack, and
- Having familial hypercholesterolemia (an inherited condition that leads to higher than normal LDL cholesterol and potentially a heart attack early in life).

Risk factors for prediabetes you can do something about

- Smoking
- Being sedentary
- Having high blood pressure
- Having high triglycerides
- Having low HDL (good) cholesterol
- Having high total LDL cholesterol, and
- Being overweight, especially if that weight is around your middle.

Of course not every overweight person is going to develop prediabetes or type 2 diabetes (many don't), but the underlying metabolic problem in prediabetes and type 2 diabetes—that is, insulin resistance—is exacerbated by being overweight.

As we explain in Chapter 2, insulin resistance means your body cells are resistant to the action of insulin. They don't let glucose in easily, so the blood glucose level tends to rise. To compensate, the pancreas makes more and more insulin. This eventually moves the glucose into the cells, but the blood insulin levels stay high. Having high insulin levels all the time spells trouble.

Being overweight makes this situation worse because the excess fat "blocks" the action of the insulin, putting added pressure on the body's ability to maintain optimal blood glucose levels.

Chapter 4

What you need to know about the metabolic syndrome

If your doctor has told you that you have high blood pressure and "a touch of sugar" (prediabetes), you probably have the metabolic syndrome. In fact, a quarter of the world's adults have metabolic syndrome. This term describes the clustering of risk factors for heart disease, including:

- Diabetes or prediabetes
- Central obesity
- High blood pressure, and
- High blood fats (triglycerides) and cholesterol.

You may also see it referred to as syndrome X or the insulin resistance syndrome.

People with the metabolic syndrome are three times as likely to have a heart attack or stroke as people without it, and they have five times more risk of developing type 2 diabetes (if it's not already present).

Insulin resistance is thought to be the reason these risk factors cluster because tests on people with the metabolic syndrome show that insulin resistance is nearly always present. Each risk factor should be treated aggressively to reduce the risk of heart disease, and in this chapter we look at how you can do this.

Risk factor 1:
Having diabetes or prediabetes

High blood glucose levels increase the tendency for blood clots to form. The resulting increased risk of heart attack is a major reason why so much effort is put into helping people with diabetes achieve optimal control of their blood glucose levels, and why all people with diabetes should be checked for the other risk factors of heart disease. But you don't need to have diabetes to be at risk—having raised fasting plasma glucose (greater than or equal to 100 mg/dL) is also a risk factor.

Here's how diabetes and prediabetes can cause inflammation and hardening of the arteries. A high level of glucose in the blood means:

- Excess glucose moves into cells lining the arteries, which causes inflammation, thickening and stiffening—the making of "hardened arteries."
- Highly reactive, charged particles called "free radicals" are formed; these destroy the machinery inside the cell, eventually causing cell death.
- Glucose sticks to cholesterol in the blood, which promotes the formation of fatty plaque and stops the body from breaking down excess cholesterol.
- Higher levels of insulin (which follow higher levels of glucose) raise blood pressure and blood fats, while lowering "good" (HDL) cholesterol levels.

Risk factor 2: Central obesity

When you put on weight, the fat can be distributed evenly all over the body or stick around the middle: what is called middle-age spread, a pot belly or a muffin top. Fat around the middle part of your body (abdominal fat) increases your risk of heart disease, high blood pressure and type 2 diabetes.

In contrast, fat on the lower part of your body, such as your hips and thighs, doesn't carry the same health risk. In fact, your body shape can be described according to your distribution of body fat as either an "apple" or a "pear" shape:

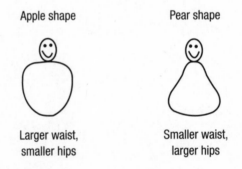

Apple shape	Pear shape
Larger waist, smaller hips	Smaller waist, larger hips

There are significant health benefits in reducing your waist measurement, particularly if you have an "apple" shape.

A healthy waist

The International Diabetes Federation has published criteria for defining the metabolic syndrome. A person with metabolic syndrome will have abdominal obesity plus at least two of the following other risk factors: high triglycerides, low HDL cholesterol, raised blood pressure and/or raised blood glucose. A basic guide to whether you have abdominal obesity is:

For people of European origin:

Men	more than 37 inches (94cm)
Women	more than 32 inches (80cm)

For ethnic South and Central Americans and people from South Asia:

Men	more than 35½ inches (90cm)
Women	more than 31½ inches (80cm)

For people from Japan:

Men	more than 35½ inches (90cm)
Women	more than 31½ inches (80cm)

These are the most recently published criteria from the International Diabetes Federation (2013).

For more information go to: www.idf.org

Risk factor 3: Having high blood pressure

High blood pressure (hypertension) is the most common heart disease risk factor. It is harmful because it demands that your heart work harder and damages your arteries.

An artery is a muscular tube. Healthy arteries can change their size to control the flow of blood. High blood pressure causes changes in the walls of arteries which makes atherosclerosis more likely to develop. Blood clots can then form, and the weakened blood vessels can easily develop a thrombosis, or rupture, and bleed.

People with diabetes should aim to keep their blood pressure under 130/85. High blood pressure is especially dangerous because it often gives no warning signs or symptoms. Your blood pressure can be high and you feel on top of the world. That's why it is important to have it checked regularly by your doctor. If it is high, there are things you can do to lower it. Just as importantly, if your blood pressure is normal, there are things you can do to keep it from becoming high.

What can you do about high blood pressure?

You can reduce your blood pressure by eating a diet rich in whole grains, fruits, vegetables and low-fat dairy products. Here are some other lifestyle characteristics that help:

- Be a nonsmoker
- Reduce your salt intake
- Achieve and maintain a healthy body weight
- Limit your alcohol intake, and
- Be active every day.

Risk factor 4: Having high blood fats (triglycerides) and cholesterol

For people with diabetes, high blood fat levels increase the risk of having a heart attack or a stroke, or developing peripheral vascular disease (for example, in the lower limbs, particularly the feet).

What causes high blood fats?

Abnormal levels of blood fats are part and parcel of the metabolic abnormalities of diabetes and prediabetes. In particular, low levels of HDL cholesterol and high triglycerides are common. For some people, genetic factors are to blame, but for the majority, diet and lifestyle factors contribute.

Blood fats

HDL cholesterol ("good" cholesterol)

HDL (high density lipoprotein) cholesterol seems to protect against heart disease because it clears cholesterol from the arteries and helps in its removal from the body. So having low levels of HDL in the blood is a risk factor for heart disease.

LDL cholesterol ("bad" cholesterol)

LDL (low density lipoprotein) cholesterol does the most damage to blood vessels. It's a red flag for heart disease. LDL cholesterol comes from the liver to the rest of the body's organs, and it can build up in the walls of blood vessels throughout the body.

Triglycerides

The blood also contains triglycerides, another type of fat linked with increased risk of heart disease. Having too much triglyceride (equal to or greater than 150 mg/dL) is often linked with having too little HDL cholesterol (high density lipoprotein). Although this can be inherited, it's most often associated with being overweight or obese.

What can you do about high blood fats?

Moderate weight loss, regular exercise and good blood glucose control will all improve blood fat levels. Dietary factors that raise triglyceride levels include eating too many high GI carbohydrates, drinking too much alcohol and not eating enough omega-3 fats. See Chapter 21, Living with prediabetes, for tips on eating a diet low in saturated fat.

Should you look out for foods that claim to be low cholesterol or cholesterol free?

Overall, it is more practical to focus on eating less saturated fat than on eating less cholesterol because saturated fats have a more powerful effect on blood cholesterol levels, and many of the foods that are high in saturated fat are also high in cholesterol anyway.

When checking food labels, use the Nutrition Facts panel to choose the food with the lower combined saturated and trans fat.

Most foods that are high in cholesterol are from animals because cholesterol is manufactured in the liver. So low cholesterol claims on rice and bread are pretty meaningless. However, some pre-processed plant-based foods have animal fats added to them when they are prepared (many cookies and cakes do), so some can contain significant amounts of cholesterol.

Chapter 5
What you need to know about diabetes management

There are certain recommendations for good health for everyone who has diabetes. Keeping your blood glucose levels as close as possible to the normal range (72–144 mg/dL) is the first step toward reducing the risk of complications. But diabetes affects the whole body, so controlling your cholesterol and blood pressure is the second step.

For some people with type 2 diabetes, all they have to do to achieve this is manage their weight, maintain a healthy eating plan and be active. Others need to take pills as well, and some may need insulin (it depends on your number of surviving beta cells).

Treating diabetes is a team effort. Ideally, on your team there will be a doctor (and possibly an endocrinologist or specialist physician), a diabetes educator, a dietitian, a podiatrist, an exercise specialist, an eye doctor and a dentist. There may also be a counselor (psychologist or psychiatrist) to help you cope with living with a chronic disease.

The most important member of your team is you, and knowledge is your best defense. Only you can make sure you know as much as possible about your diabetes, and only you can act on the advice that you are given.

So, what do you need to aim for?

- Hemoglobin A1c (2–3 month average blood glucose)—under 7 percent, or 53 mmol/mol
- Blood glucose levels 72–144 mg/dL
- Blood pressure—under 120/80 mm Hg
- Cholesterol—under 100 mg/dL
- Healthy weight
- Healthy eating plan
- Regular exercise
- Regular eye checks, and
- Regular foot examinations.

If the combination of weight loss (if necessary), a healthy diet, physical activity and medication delivers near normal blood glucose levels, your diabetes is well managed and your risk of complications is much lower. Unfortunately, it doesn't mean that your diabetes has gone away.

Working with a healthcare team

Working with a healthcare team is the best way you can avoid the serious complications that diabetes can cause. That's the clear message from numerous studies of people with diabetes in recent years. And that's why you'll find the rest of this chapter is rather full of lists (sorry!).

What we have tried to do is give you as comprehensive a picture as possible of the sorts of tests and checkups you need, and how often you need them. If you find that you can't talk comfortably with anyone on your healthcare team, or that they don't give you the tests or information you need, go and find someone who will give you the care you deserve—and the answers to your questions. Don't hesitate to take this book (or a photocopy of the relevant pages) along with you to your appointments to refer to if it will help.

Seeing your family doctor

In most cases it's the family doctor who diagnoses diabetes and plays the central role in coordinating care. It is essential that you are happy with your doctor and feel comfortable talking to him or her, and that he or she understands what needs to be done.

What your doctor needs to do

Initial visits

- Give you general information about your diabetes so that you understand what it is and why effectively managing it is so important
- Measure your weight, height and waist
- Check your blood pressure
- Order blood tests to check your:
  - hemoglobin A1c (HbA1c) level, which is a measure of the average level of glucose in your blood over the last 2–3 months
  - liver function
  - cholesterol and triglyceride levels
  - creatinine level to see whether your kidneys are working properly
- Ask you to do a urine test to check for early signs of kidney problems
- Refer you to a diabetes educator to give you more information about how you can manage your diabetes yourself
- Refer you to a registered dietitian to help you lose weight if you need to and determine the quantity and type of food to eat, and
- Consider referring you to an endocrinologist, podiatrist, exercise specialist and/or other member of the diabetes management team, depending on your particular needs.

Even if your diabetes and any associated complications are being well managed, it is a good idea to have a checkup with your doctor every 3–6 months.

Checkups

- Check your blood pressure
- Check your weight
- Measure your waist circumference
- Order a blood test to check your hemoglobin A1c levels. HbA1c levels need to be checked every 3–6 months if you are using insulin, and every 6–12 months if you are not using insulin
- Check your cholesterol/triglyceride levels if they are above normal
- Help you set goals for managing your diabetes and discuss your progress toward achieving them, and
- Do a basic foot examination (every 6 months).

Each year

- Discuss how well you are managing your diabetes
- Check your cholesterol/triglyceride levels
- Ask you to do a urine test to check for early signs of kidney problems
- Discuss referral to an ophthalmologist or optometrist to have your eyes examined for early signs of retinopathy, and
- Refer you to an endocrinologist, diabetes educator, dietitian, podiatrist, exercise specialist and/or other health professionals as required.

**Do you need to see an endocrinologist
or a specialist diabetes physician?**

Your doctor may refer you to an endocrinologist or specialist physician if:

- Your hemoglobin A1c level is persistently over 8 percent, or 183 mg/dL
- You have been in the hospital for a diabetes-related problem
- You have other health problems associated with your diabetes, and/or
- You are pregnant or thinking of becoming pregnant.

Seeing a diabetes educator

Diabetes educators are healthcare professionals who specialize in helping people with diabetes stay healthy. Depending on your specific situation, your diabetes educator will work with you to develop a plan to help you manage your diabetes.

When should you see a diabetes educator?

- When you are first diagnosed with diabetes
- For an annual checkup, and
- If you change the way you manage your diabetes. For example, if you change from managing your diabetes simply by following a healthy lifestyle to taking pills, or from taking pills to using insulin.
  It's also recommended you have a follow-up meeting if:
- Your HbA1c is persistently above 8 percent (183 mg/dL), and/or
- You are pregnant.

Finding a diabetes educator

Your doctor may refer you to a diabetes educator, or you can find one through the American Association of Diabetes Educators (AADE), details of which are found in the Resources section of this book.

What a diabetes management plan may cover

- How to monitor your blood glucose levels and use the results to improve your diabetes management
- How to prevent, detect and treat high and low blood glucose readings and manage on sick days
- How to use your medications effectively on sick days
- How to manage your blood glucose, cholesterol and blood pressure levels
- What to do to reduce the risk of developing long-term complications of diabetes, including knowledge of risk-factor screening recommendations, ideal targets and personal targets
- Tips for communicating effectively with your diabetes healthcare team and negotiating your way through the healthcare system, and
- Advice on adapting your work, family and social life to live well with diabetes.

Seeing a dietitian

A registered dietitian can provide specific advice tailored to your current eating habits and food preferences and will work with you to set realistic and achievable goals. They will help you understand the relationship between food and health and guide you toward making dietary choices that optimize your health.

When should you see a dietitian?

- When you are first diagnosed with diabetes, and possibly every 4 weeks for the first 3 months after you have been diagnosed, and then every 6–12 months after that
- Whenever you change the way you manage your diabetes
- If you are overweight
- If you are pregnant or thinking of becoming pregnant
- If your HbA1c is persistently above 8 percent (183 mg/dL)
- If you have high blood pressure, cholesterol or triglycerides
- If you have diabetes and another condition such as heart disease, kidney impairment, celiac disease or osteoporosis, and
- If you have problems managing your diabetes.

Finding a dietitian

Dietitians have professionally recognized qualifications in human nutrition. They practice as individual professionals and are available through most public hospitals and in private practice.

Seeing a podiatrist

Blood glucose levels that are high for long periods of time can damage nerves in the legs and feet, causing numbness or a burning sensation. If this happens, you can injure your feet without knowing it. If your diabetes is poorly managed, the blood vessels can become thick, rigid and narrow. Damage to the blood flow in your feet and legs can lead to problems such as infection, ulcers and even gangrene. It's essential that people with diabetes practice good footcare, hence, the recommendation to include a podiatrist on your healthcare team.

When should you see a podiatrist?

Annually for a routine diabetes foot check, and more often if you:

- Have a foot ulcer or have had one in the past
- Have had part or all of a foot amputated
- Have neuropathy (damage to the nerves in your feet)
- Have been told that you have problems with blood flow to your feet
- Have corns or calluses or other foot problems, including injuries that are slow to heal
- Have any problems or pain walking
- Have trouble finding shoes that fit you, and/or
- Can't look after your own footcare (can't reach your feet or have poor eyesight).

Seeing an exercise specialist

Did you know that you can improve your blood glucose levels, your blood fat levels and your body weight simply by being more active? A physiotherapist, exercise physiologist or certified personal trainer can help you work out a program to improve your overall physical fitness, increase your total muscle mass and decrease your body fat.

When might you think about seeing an exercise specialist?

- When you are first diagnosed with diabetes
- If your HbA1c is persistently above 8 percent or 64 mmol/mol
- If you have high blood pressure, cholesterol or triglycerides
- If you have diabetes and another condition (such as problems with your heart or circulation)
- If you are overweight, and/or
- If you are having problems managing your diabetes.

Seeing an eye specialist

Everyone with diabetes is advised to have regular eye examinations with an eye specialist or optometrist because early treatment can prevent the visual loss that can be part and parcel of diabetes.

Seeing a dentist

If you have diabetes, you are at greater risk of developing gum disease, including gingivitis and periodontitis (sore bleeding gums). Some studies also suggest that because gum disease is an infection, it can contribute to higher blood glucose levels. So it is important to keep your regular dental appointments. When you visit, remind your dentist that you have diabetes.

4 steps to preventing gum disease

- Brush your teeth twice a day and floss once a day
- Visit your dentist every 6 months for a checkup and cleaning to remove the build-up of tartar from areas your brush can't reach
- Manage your blood glucose levels, and
- Do not smoke—people who smoke are four times more likely to develop gum disease than people who don't.

Seeing a counselor

A psychologist or psychiatrist can help you make positive changes to your life that may make managing diabetes easier.

When might you think about seeing a counselor?

- If you suffer from stress because of your diabetes
- You are depressed or anxious, and/or
- You are having problems managing your diabetes.

Consumer health organizations such as diabetes associations can also play an important part in helping you manage diabetes, through membership, meetings, magazines and subsidized products.

Unfortunately, some people, despite their best efforts, find their diabetes difficult to manage and can't get the control they want. And again, despite hard work, some people still develop complications. This can be pretty discouraging. Just remember that if you do the best job you can day by day, you will reduce the risk of complications later on and slow the progress of complications that may be just beginning.

What happens if diabetes is not managed well?

If blood glucose levels are not well managed, you can suffer damage to the blood vessels in the heart, legs, brain, eyes and kidneys. That's why heart attacks, leg amputations, strokes, blindness and kidney failure are more common in people with diabetes. Diabetes can also damage the nerves in your feet, causing pain and irritation in your feet and numbness and loss of sensation.

High blood pressure, high cholesterol, smoking and being overweight or obese can also lead to diabetes complications, especially damage to the blood vessels, which can, in turn, cause heart attacks and stroke and affect the circulation to the legs. That's why it's very important to deal with these problems to stay healthy.

Some of the things you'll need to deal with

1. Health professionals

The job of health professionals (e.g., general practitioner, diabetes educator, dietitian, endocrinologist) is to help you look after your diabetes yourself. If you think your healthcare providers are not treating you with the respect you deserve, talk to them openly about your feelings. If this does not lead to any improvement, politely ask to be referred to someone else.

2. Telling others

Who needs to know that you have diabetes? There is no need to go around shouting to the world that you have diabetes; on the other hand, there is no need to be ashamed of it either. So how do you decide who to tell? While there are no hard and fast rules, these ideas might help you make up your mind.

First, consider how often you see a person and what you do together when you meet. If you are to share a meal, why hide the fact that you have diabetes and need to check your blood glucose level and take insulin or medication? You have nothing to be ashamed of—go ahead, tell them.

On the other hand, if you just run in to them from time to time and all you do is chat briefly, do they really need to know?

Classmates, coworkers, employers, or other people you see every day may need to know more. For example, if you take insulin or pills that may make your blood glucose go low, you should tell your colleagues, because you may have to duck out and have a quick snack in the middle of something important—a game, a meeting, a class.

If you operate machinery or perform tasks that may put your or someone else's life at risk, you are morally obligated to let those who work with you know.

However, if you manage your diabetes or prediabetes with a healthy lifestyle, you probably do not need to tell your colleagues. If they ask you, though, it's wise to tell the truth.

3. The diet police

Let's face it—most people know, or have known, someone who has diabetes. If it was someone who was diagnosed just 20 years ago, chances are they were advised to avoid sugar in their diet as much as possible—this was the standard recommendation for all people with diabetes for most of the 20th century. That's why many people equate the management of diabetes with the avoidance of all sugar. But research has proven that people with diabetes can eat the same amount of sugar as the average person without compromising blood glucose levels. Of course "empty calories"—whatever the source: sugar, starch, fat or alcohol—won't keep the engine running smoothly. "Moderation in all things" is a good motto.

How many times have you been asked "should you be eating that?" by an observer? While they have good intentions, it can be downright irritating. And wrong.

Beyond irritation, it can become dangerous if well-meaning individuals try to stop you having a sweet or drink when you are having low blood sugar—there are more than a few stories of people having a potentially lifesaving "treat" snatched out of their hand!

But what can you do? If you are not having low blood sugar, you can politely explain that the recommendation to avoid sugar was based on experiments on dogs in the 1920s. We have known for the past 30 years that sugar does not upset blood glucose levels any more than a typical slice of bread.

Knowing why and how to look after yourself is very important, and once you are informed, you can enlighten other people about the modern management of diabetes.

PART 2:

What *you* can do to take control of the things in your life you can change

Chapter 6
5 steps to managing diabetes

The way you live will have a major impact on your diabetes, especially on your blood glucose levels. There are 5 key areas of your lifestyle/health to address in looking after diabetes. Not all the steps will apply to you. For example, if you don't need to lose weight or you don't smoke or drink alcohol, you may want to skip some of the chapters in this section.

Step 1: Eat a healthy, balanced diet

Of course everybody should maintain a healthy, balanced eating plan. But it's not negotiable for people managing diabetes. In fact, many people can manage their diabetes simply by choosing the right kinds and amounts of foods (along with being active every day).

Step 2: Be active every day

We were made to move. But we don't do much of it these days in our push-button, "let your fingers do the walking" world. Too many of us lead busy, but sedentary, desk-bound, commuting lives. We relax in front of the TV and exercise infrequently or not at all.

Regular moderate physical activity is essential for managing diabetes and for reducing heart disease risk. Doing housework or gardening, or going for a brisk walk on a regular basis, all count toward increasing your activity level. Boosting them with regular, moderate-intensity exercise sessions can help you manage your blood glucose levels and reduce the risk of diabetes complications and heart disease.

How does it work? Exercise and activity increase glucose and insulin uptake and can:

- Help lower your blood pressure
- Reduce your heart attack risk
- Reduce your insulin requirements
- Help you stop smoking
- Help you manage your weight
- Increase your levels of good (HDL) cholesterol
- Help keep your bones and joints strong
- Improve your mood
- Ease depression
- Increase your stamina, and
- Increase your flexibility.

Step 3: Manage your weight

Besides making diabetes harder to control, being overweight puts you at a much greater risk of heart disease and high blood pressure. Being overweight also interferes with sleep because fat around the neck area and abdomen induces a form of snoring called sleep apnea, which means you could become tired and cranky as well. So losing a little weight, or at least stabilizing it if you are on the heavy side, has to be a priority.

The good news is you don't have to be "the biggest loser." Setting achievable weight loss goals is the key. Research suggests that there are significant health benefits even when you lose just 5–10 percent of your body weight. For example, if you weigh 220 lbs, losing around 12–22 lbs over 12–24 weeks is realistic and safe—and enough to improve your health. If you achieve this and maintain the weight loss long term, your risk of developing other chronic diseases and the complications of diabetes will be substantially reduced.

In Chapter 18 we look more closely at body energy balance and what it takes to lose weight. We outline some workable approaches to weight management, setting realistic goals for body weight, and developing habits that may help you manage your weight.

Step 4: Don't smoke. If you do, quit

Smoking is most often associated with lung and other cancers, but it may also increase the risk of developing diabetes, and many of the common complications of diabetes.

And did you know that smokers have more than twice the heart attack risk of nonsmokers and are much more likely to die if they suffer a heart attack? In fact smoking is the most preventable risk factor for heart disease. Research has shown that smoking just one cigarette reduces the body's ability to use insulin by 15 percent! After a cigarette it takes 10–12 hours before the insulin resistance starts to improve.

In Chapter 19 we look at smoking and diabetes.

Step 5: Limit your consumption of alcohol

Like most things in life, moderation is the key. One or two drinks each day may actually help prevent or delay the development of diabetes, and some of its more common complications, by decreasing insulin resistance. It may also decrease the risk of developing heart disease, by providing small amounts of powerful antioxidants and thinning the blood. On the other hand, excessive amounts of alcohol may increase the risk of prediabetes and diabetes by contributing to weight gain—particularly if your drinking goes along with eating high calorie foods.

If you have diabetes or prediabetes, it's important to limit your consumption of alcohol to no more than one standard drink a day if you are a woman and two standard drinks if you are a man.

In Chapter 20 we look in more detail at alcohol and diabetes.

STEP 1:
EAT A HEALTHY, BALANCED DIET

In the following chapters we show you how you can eat a healthy balanced diet that will keep you feeling fuller for longer, help keep your blood glucose levels on an even keel and reduce your risk of complications by helping you manage your blood pressure and blood fat levels.

Chapter 7
Just tell me what to eat

There is no absolute "right" way to eat to manage diabetes. Only you can really tell what eating plan suits you best: you know what works for you and how you feel.

It's tempting to simply try to write out lists of "what to eat" and "what not to eat." But it just can't be done. Take sugar, for instance. Any self-respecting person with diabetes would put it on the taboo list. Wouldn't they? Well, not necessarily. Eating well if you have diabetes isn't about good foods and bad foods, eating this and avoiding that. It's about enjoying *all* foods for nourishment and pleasure, just coupled with a knowledge of and respect for your body's needs (and if you're wondering how sugar fits in, check Chapter 15.)

There are three aspects of eating well for diabetes management:

- What you eat
- How much you eat, and
- When you eat.

Why what you eat is important

Your health and vitality depend on the quality of the food your body receives. Besides protein, fat and carbohydrate, you need vitamins to help your body convert food into fuel, minerals to carry oxygen in your blood, antioxidants to boost your defense system and phytochemicals to prevent disease (just to name a few).

Why how much you eat is important

Achieving or maintaining a healthy weight will help you manage your blood glucose. Too many calories, whether they are carbohydrate, protein or fat, will increase your body weight. Too much carbohydrate will raise your blood glucose levels. The trick is to find the amount and combination of healthy foods that's right for you.

Why when you eat is important

Eating regularly almost inevitably improves blood glucose levels, and there are probably several reasons for this. Most meal plans for diabetes include three meals each day. They may include snacks as well—there are no hard and fast rules about how many times a day you will need to eat.

10 key dietary recommendations

Remember what we said at the beginning of this chapter: there isn't any one diet for everybody with diabetes. What this means is that you actually have a great deal of flexibility in the overall make-up of your eating plan. It's a matter of discovering what suits you best while fitting within these recommendations:

- Choose nutritious carbohydrate foods with a low GI as your staples, and limit your intake of high GI carbohydrate-containing foods
- Be aware of how much carbohydrate you eat
- Get plenty of fiber in your diet
- Limit foods that are high in saturated fat
- Eat lean protein foods to suit your appetite
- Eat fish once or twice a week: if you are vegetarian, make sure you focus on including foods that contain quality proteins and are good sources of omega-3 fats

- Use monounsaturated fats (such as olive oil)
- Eat plenty of fruit and vegetables every day
- Moderate your salt intake, and
- Limit your alcohol intake.

From food to fuel:
A little bit of basic nutrition

The human body truly is a marvellous machine. It converts the energy found in food in a zillion different processes, from the micro (molecular change) to the macro (you taking a step) level. Your body needs food for energy, just like cars need gas. However, unlike cars, which can run on just one type of fuel, your body needs three different fuel sources: protein, fat and carbohydrate (we can burn alcohol too, but it's an optional extra).

The energy available from these three fuels ranges from 4 calories per gram of protein or carbohydrate to 9 calories per gram of fat. It's kind of like standard fuel compared with super high octane. You get the most mileage from fat. (Unfortunately, though, most of us don't drive our bodies nearly as much as we drive our cars.)

There is a fuel hierarchy, too. That is, the body follows a particular order for burning the fuels you take in. If you drink, alcohol is at the top of the list because your body has no place to store unused alcohol. Excess protein comes next (because we can store only a little); carbohydrate is third in line (we can store some); and fat comes off last (we have unlimited storage space for fat). In practice, the fuel mix is usually a combination of carbohydrate and fat in varying proportions. After meals, the fuel is predominantly carbohydrate, and between meals it is mainly fat. In Chapter 8, we cover nutrition basics and take a look at protein, fat and carbs.

Water

Water is an often forgotten essential nutrient. It is critical for every bodily function. But for a lot of people, water is not part of their daily diet. We may not need the popularly recommended 8 glasses a day, but we all need some, and if we smoke, drink alcohol, consume caffeine or are physically active, we need more.

Drinking water is a habit, and it's one of the habits we want you to have. To get started, make it available. Whatever type of water you like—filtered, bottled or plain old tap water—make sure it's in front of you all the time. Then make a habit of drinking it.

The color of your urine tells you how well hydrated you are:

- Clear or very pale indicates good hydration, and
- Darker colored (except for first thing in the morning) suggests dehydration.

Chapter 8

Nutrition basics: What you need to know about protein, fat and carbs

Protein foods

Protein is part of every cell, and is therefore vital in the growth and repair of tissues throughout your body. It is made up of amino acids, which are the building blocks for the body. They form your hair, skin, muscles, hormones, blood cells, etc. Protein can also be used as a fuel. Indeed, any excess beyond your immediate needs (for amino acids) is quickly converted to energy.

Protein is found in lots of plant and animal foods. The foods with the most protein are meat (beef, pork, lamb, chicken, turkey), fish and seafood. Dairy products such as cheese (especially cottage cheese), milk and yogurt are also rich sources. For vegetarians, legumes including soybeans and their products (tofu), nuts and grains are significant sources. Protein foods, especially meat, are also rich sources of micronutrients such as iron, zinc and vitamin B12, and fish is a source of omega-3 fats.

Protein and blood glucose

Protein does not directly affect your blood glucose levels, but just like carbohydrate, it does stimulate secretion of significant amounts of insulin. Up to half the protein you eat will eventually be converted to glucose via a process called "gluconeogenesis" (which literally means the creation of new glucose). However, after you eat a protein-rich meal, your glucose concentrations do not rise and fall in any marked way because your body balances the rate of glucose production with the rate of glucose burning.

How much do you need?

As you grow, so do your protein needs. That's why children, adolescents and pregnant women need more protein than healthy, full-grown adults. It's the same scenario if you are recovering from an injury (healing burns or wounds), from a major illness, or repairing or building muscles (as athletes or weekend warriors do)—your protein needs are greater.

When your blood glucose levels are high, as they are in diabetes, there is an increase in your protein turnover, and this in turn increases your body's protein needs slightly. However, because most people already consume much more protein than they need, eating even more protein is not usually recommended.

Most people with diabetes can stick with their regular protein intake: it usually provides about 15–20 percent of their total energy intake. As long as you have enough food to eat, you will be getting enough protein because it is so widely available in the food supply.

Fat

You're about to butter your toast at breakfast and then you hesitate. Would margarine be better? Maybe you shouldn't use anything at all? But dry toast isn't very appealing.

In 1927, Harvard Medical School Professor Elliot P. Joslin wrote: "With an excess of fat, diabetes begins, and from an excess of fat, diabetics die." Although Joslin wrote that nearly 90 years ago, he was right. Excess body fat definitely contributes to the development of diabetes. The increasing prevalence of both obesity and diabetes supports that. And there is good evidence linking a high saturated fat intake to the complications of diabetes. But is a low-fat diet the answer?

What's the problem with fat?

One problem with fat is the amount we eat (sometimes without knowing it). Fat provides a lot of calories and is the least satiating nutrient. This is great for someone who's starving, but it's a real disadvantage for those of us who constantly verge on eating too much. Fat provides 9 calories per gram—more than twice the energy of protein or carbohydrate. And the main form in which our bodies store those extra calories is (you guessed it)—fat. Indeed, scientists can tell what sort of fat you've been eating by analysing a slice of your body fat.

Another problem is heart disease. As we explained earlier, people with diabetes have a greatly increased risk of cardiovascular disease—heart disease and stroke are 2–3 times more likely in people with diabetes than in those without, and almost 70 percent of people with type 2 diabetes die of cardiovascular disease. High levels of LDL (bad) and total cholesterol are a known risk factor for cardiovascular disease, and reducing total fat—and in particular saturated fat—lowers both total and LDL cholesterol, and therefore decreases this risk.

Whatever the fat content of your diet (low or moderate), the type of fat you eat matters—monounsaturated fats (found in nuts, seeds, olive oil, avocado, etc.) should dominate. Eating more fat from these sources gives you a nutritional profile more like a Mediterranean diet, which will also help you lower your triglyceride levels and LDL (bad) cholesterol. However, you need to remember that the Mediterranean diet carries a risk of weight gain (if it's not calorie controlled) and, in the long run, may not benefit your glycemic control.

What happens when we eat fat?

The digestion of fat is a slow process compared with the digestion of protein and carbs—it doesn't really begin until the fat reaches your small intestine. Here bile works rather like detergent in the dishwasher, breaking up fats into small droplets that are cleaved apart by an enzyme from the pancreas. About 3 hours after eating, the digested fat is fully absorbed. Once absorbed, the fat circulates in your bloodstream as triglycerides.

What are triglycerides?

Triglycerides are the white fat you see on meat. They come from fats we eat in foods, but they are also made in the body from excess carbohydrate, and they circulate in our bloodstream after meals. Calories that are in excess of our body's needs can be converted into triglycerides and transported to fat cells to be stored. Excess triglycerides in the blood are a common characteristic of diabetes and have a bad effect on metabolism. They also, of course, contribute to the increased risk of heart disease, stroke and liver disease.

Triglyceride levels rise gradually after a meal, and in a person who doesn't have diabetes, they return to pre-meal levels after 4–6 hours. But in people with type 2 diabetes, the clearance of triglycerides from the circulation is delayed, and having high levels in your bloodstream for a long time is harmful. Here's what high triglycerides do:

- They impair insulin's action, thus suppressing glucose uptake and use by muscles, which means that glucose hangs around in the bloodstream

- They stimulate the liver to make more glucose, raising blood glucose levels even further
- They cause the liver to form fatty particles that are toxic to blood vessels
- They accumulate in the liver and cause "fatty liver," and
- They impair insulin secretion (possibly by accumulating in the pancreas and impairing beta cell function).

All in all, this means a high fat meal can be pretty bad news for your diabetes.

What fat is that?

Although all fats provide about the same number of calories per gram (and so are theoretically as fattening as each other), there are differences in the nature of the fatty acids they contain, and those differences have major implications for your health.

Fats are broadly classified into three groups—polyunsaturated, monounsaturated and saturated. The classification is based on the chemical structure of the fat and the type of fatty acid that is dominant.

What's a fatty acid?

A fatty acid is a chain of carbon and hydrogen atoms bonded together. Most fats contain three fatty acids joined by a glycerol backbone to form one fat molecule or triglyceride.

Polyunsaturated fats

These are found in seed oils, seafood, nuts and seeds. They are liquid in nature. The most common examples are safflower, sunflower, soybean and cottonseed oils, which are rich in omega-6 fats. These fats all have cholesterol-lowering properties, but like saturated fats, we can eat too much of them.

Omega-3 fats are another form of polyunsaturated fat. Very long chain forms are found in significant quantities in fish, and a shorter form is found in some plant oils, including canola, flaxseed and walnut oils. They can reduce your risk of cardiovascular disease too, mostly by reducing your triglyceride levels. Many of us don't get the recommended quantities of the omega-3 fats we need.

Monounsaturated fats

These are found in virtually all edible fats, but canola and olive oils, margarines made from these oils, nuts and avocados are particularly rich sources. These fats can protect you against heart disease and lower LDL (bad) cholesterol levels. Although olive oil doesn't have a lot of omega-3 fatty acids (which are good), it has the advantage of not providing a lot of omega-6 fats. It also has the longest history of safe and healthy use and is rich in antioxidants if it is "cold pressed" (look for "first cold pressing" on the label).

Saturated fats

These are solid at room temperature—the more saturated fatty acids there are in the fat, the harder it is at room temperature. Saturated fats are generally not good for our health. They decrease the effectiveness of insulin, increase LDL cholesterol levels and increase heart disease risk. Eating foods rich in certain saturated fats promotes the formation of too much LDL cholesterol in our blood. High blood cholesterol is strongly associated with heart disease risk.

Drippings (fat from beef and lamb), lard (fat from pork), butter and cream are largely saturated fat.

Trans fats

These occur naturally in a few foods like butter, cheese and meat. They are also formed in food manufacturing when vegetable oils are processed and made more solid. Think of them as saturated fats because they damage the body in a similar way. Commercial baked goods (such as crackers, cookies and cakes) and fried foods (such as doughnuts and french fries) are likely to contain trans fats.

How much fat do you need?

Not everyone has to cut down on their fat intake. If you are a healthy weight now (and have no problems maintaining it), you may not need to reduce the amount of fat you eat at all. (It is interesting to note that breastfed infants get 50–60 percent of their energy intake as fat?)

So how much fat is enough? And how much is too much?

Minimum: The World Health Organization recommends that men get at least 15 percent of their energy (calories) from fat and women of reproductive age get at least 20 percent.

Maximum: The upper level for adults is 35 percent of their energy. This translates to about 50–60g of fat daily for a sedentary adult, not more than 15–20g of which should be saturated.

We all need some fat because:

- It is part of all our cell membranes
- It is a carrier of fat soluble vitamins A, D, E and K and many antioxidants
- It is an integral part of many hormones

- It is an energy source, and
- It provides insulation, for warmth and protection of vital organs like the kidneys.

The absolutely essential fatty acids that we must get in our diet—because our body can't make them—are alpha-linolenic acid (ALA) and linoleic acid (LA). ALA is an omega-3 fat found in linseed, canola, walnuts and some dark green leafy vegetables. LA is an omega-6 fat found in corn, safflower and sunflower oils.

Getting rid of bad fats

Saturated and trans fats are some fats that we all need to eat less of. An intake of less than 10 percent of your total calories per day from saturated fats and less than 2 percent from trans fats is what's recommended. For an average diet of 2,000 calories, this means a maximum of 15–20g of saturated fat per day.

Choosing the good fats

A healthy balance of fats means including *some* polyunsaturated oils which are rich in omega-6 fats (such as corn, soybean and safflower oils) and more sources of omega-3 (such as fish, canola, flaxseeds, walnuts, pecans and soybeans). A monounsaturated fat such as olive oil is a good general oil to use.

Carbohydrate

Carbohydrate is a part of food. Starch is a carbohydrate; so are sugars and most types of fiber. Starches and sugars are nature's reserves, created by energy from the sun, carbon dioxide and water. Carbohydrate comes mainly from plant foods, such as cereal grains, fruits, vegetables and legumes (peas and beans). Milk and yogurt also contain carbohydrate, in the form of milk sugar (lactose). The following foods are good sources of carbohydrate:

- **Cereals and grains** such as wheat, rice, corn, oats, barley, bread and breakfast cereals. These are rich in starch and vary from 20–85 percent carbohydrate by weight
- **Legumes** such as cannellini beans, lentils, chickpeas and split peas are also rich in starch and contain 55–65 percent carbohydrate
- **Some root vegetables**, such as potatoes, sweet potatoes, yams, taro and cassava, contain 10–25 percent starch. Most other vegetables (broccoli, zucchini, tomatoes, etc.) contain no starch and only minor amounts of natural sugars
- **Fruits** range from 5–15 percent carbohydrate (berries to bananas, respectively) in the form of sugars. Bananas are the only ones containing some starch in the ripe state
- **Milk** is around 5 percent carbohydrate, in the form of the sugar, lactose
- **Honey** is 75 percent sugars (fructose, glucose, sucrose), and
- **Processed foods** may contain large amounts of added sugars. Examples are cookies (35 percent sugars) and chocolate (56 percent sugars).

Sugars, starches and dietary fibers

Sugars: the simplest form of carbohydrate is a single sugar molecule called a monosaccharide (mono meaning one, saccharide meaning sweet). Glucose is a monosaccharide that occurs in food (as glucose itself, and as the building block of starch); it is the most common source of fuel for the cells of the human body.

When two monosaccharides join, the result is a disaccharide (di meaning two). Sucrose, or common table sugar, is a disaccharide, as is lactose, the sugar in milk. As the number of monosaccharides in the chain increases, the carbohydrate becomes less sweet. Maltodextrins are oligosaccharides (oligo meaning a few) that are five or six glucose residues long; they are often used as a food ingredient. They taste only slightly sweet.

Starches: at least half the glucose in your body comes from starches in your food. Starches are long chains of sugar molecules joined together like pearls in a necklace. They are called polysaccharides (poly meaning many). Starches are not sweet-tasting at all. When you eat starches, your body breaks them down into glucose units, rather like chopping up the string of pearls at random. Amylose and amylopectin are common forms of starch.

Dietary fibers: these are usually large carbohydrate molecules containing many different sorts of monosaccharides. They are different from starches and sugars in that they do not get broken down by human digestive enzymes. Fibers reach the large intestine without change. Once there, bacteria begin to ferment and break them down.

Different fibers have different physical and chemical properties. Soluble fibers can be dissolved in water. Some soluble fibers are very viscous (syrupy) when they are in solution, so they slow down the speed of digestion. Other fibers, such as cellulose, are insoluble (do not dissolve in water) and do not directly affect the speed of digestion.

Why do you need it?

Carbohydrate is the body's main energy source and an essential source of fuel for the brain—which is the most energy-demanding organ in your body. Unlike muscle cells, which can burn either fat or carbohydrate, the brain cannot burn fat. Strictly speaking, humans can "get by" on as little as 50g of carbohydrate a day. But your muscles and brain will complain: you'll tire easily and feel "headachy." In time, your body might adjust, but nutritionally speaking, it's not ideal.

If you fast for 24 hours or decide to limit your carbohydrate intake, your brain relies first on the stores of carbohydrate in the liver, but within hours these are used up, and the liver begins creating glucose from non-carbohydrate sources (including amino acids from muscle tissue). It has only a limited ability to do this, however.

We now know that any shortfall in glucose availability affects brain function, and not in a good way. People with diabetes have first-hand experience of this if they've ever suffered hypoglycemia or low blood sugar—confusion, trembling, dizziness, nausea, incoherent rambling speech and lack of coordination are what happen when the brain and central nervous system are not getting enough glucose.

How much do you need?

The current recommendation from health authorities around the world is to aim to meet 45–60 percent of your energy requirements with carbohydrate foods. However, you need to take into account your personal food preferences and your overall eating patterns when working out how much carbohydrate is right for you. Also, a person's total energy requirements differ according to age, gender, body size and activity level.

How much carbohydrate should you eat?

Having diabetes doesn't mean that you need less carbohydrate than anyone else. It just means that how much you need takes more careful thought. Because of your relative insufficiency of insulin, too much carbohydrate may be bad for your glycemic control . See Part 3 for details on daily carb needs.

What we now know is that not all carbs were created equal. In the next chapter we cover various approaches to the diet for diabetes, including carb exchanges and carb counting, and explain what's wrong with a low carb diet. And in Chapter 10 we look at carbohydrate quality and the glycemic index (GI).

Chapter 9

Carb quantity: Coming to grips with the eating plan for diabetes

Carbohydrate is an important part of your diet: it helps keep your body sensitive to insulin and gives you stamina. It is also the only part of food that directly affects your blood glucose levels. As we have explained, when you eat carbohydrate foods, they are broken down into glucose and this lifts your blood glucose levels. Your body responds by releasing insulin into the blood. The insulin clears the glucose from the blood, moving it into your muscles, where it is used for energy, so the blood glucose level returns to normal. This is why dietary tools for people with diabetes focus on carbohydrate. Dietary approaches to a healthy way of eating for diabetes today will usually incorporate guidance regarding how much, what type and when to eat carbohydrate.

The two main approaches to quantifying carbohydrate in the diet are:

- A carbohydrate exchange system, or
- Carbohydrate counting.

Carbohydrate exchanges

With the exchange approach, carbohydrate foods are identified in specific quantities known as exchanges or portions. You then eat a certain number of carbohydrate exchanges for each meal over the day. The aim is to promote consistency in the amount of carbohydrate you eat from day to day.

A carbohydrate exchange is an amount of food typically containing 10 or 15g of carbohydrate (depending on where you live) such as:

- 1 slice of bread
- 1 cup milk, and
- 1 small piece of fruit.

Carbohydrate exchange lists are available that detail serving sizes for different types of breads, biscuits, breakfast cereals, fruit, starchy vegetables and dairy products that provide 15 grams of carbohydrate. A dietitian will then recommend a certain number of carbohydrate exchanges for each meal over the course of the day.

Problems with carb exchanges

Although this system has been widely used around the world, many people with diabetes have difficulty using it. It can be a tricky concept to get your head around at first, and estimating carbohydrate exchange amounts in a plate of food isn't easy, particularly if the food is unfamiliar, or doesn't fit readily into one of the carbohydrate exchange groups. Take a lavash wrap filled with crumbed pieces of chicken, chickpeas and salad, for example. Where do you start!

Another problem with the exchange system is that it doesn't take into account the physical nature of the carbohydrate in a food and what actually happens in your body when you eat it. It assumes that the glycemic potency of each carbohydrate exchange is the same.

Carbohydrate counting

Carbohydrate counting means what it says—simply counting the actual number of grams of carbohydrate in the foods you eat by using food composition tables, the nutrition labels on food packages or an experienced estimate.

With this method (and with the exchange system) you really need to get familiar with household measures like cups and tablespoons and have a set of kitchen scales at home. You also need to learn how to interpret food labels, and how to access other sources of information (like websites, apps and books) on the carbohydrate content of foods.

Memorizing the percentage carbohydrate of common foods such as rice, bread, dry cereal, fruit, potato and milk can also help you judge your carbohydrate intake. For example, bread averages 50 percent carbohydrate, so if you know the weight of the bread you're eating, you'll know you have half that amount of carbohydrate, in grams.

With a system of carbohydrate counting your carbohydrate choices aren't limited by the extent of whichever exchange list you use, so it does allow more dietary freedom. In this regard it's a good idea to be mindful of basic nutrition principles.

Problems with carb counting

Like carbohydrate exchanges, carb counting does not take into account differences in the type of carbohydrate. The secret to the diet for diabetes is not just the *quantity* but also the *type* of carbohydrate you eat. And that's where the GI comes in.

What you need to know about low carbohydrate diets

Low carbohydrate diets are either high protein or high fat or both. They cannot be anything else because you have to get your energy from something (and alcohol in large amounts, the only other energy source for humans, won't keep you alive for long).

There are at least two variations of carbohydrate intake on a low carbohydrate diet. There are those that are:

- *Very low* in carbohydrate, containing less than 100g carbohydrate per day, or
- *Extremely low* in carbohydrate, containing as little as 20–50g carbohydrate per day (also known as ketogenic diets).

The "extremely low" variation is often found in the "kick start" phase of popular diet books. It is not recommended for anyone with diabetes.

Some problems you can have if you don't have enough carbohydrate in your diet

- Muscle fatigue, causing moderate exercise to be an enormous effort
- Insufficient fiber intake, causing constipation
- Headaches and tiredness due to low blood glucose levels, and
- Bad breath due to the breakdown products of fat (ketones).

A major concern, however, with low carb diets is the possibility of eating too much saturated fat. The long-term effect would be an increase in your LDL (bad) cholesterol.

Also, your intake of fruit, vegetables and cereal grains would be low on a low carb diet, so you probably need to take vitamin and mineral supplements, particularly to meet folate and fiber requirements.

Low carbohydrate diets may also be high in protein. There is a growing body of evidence to support moderate carbohydrate, higher protein diets for weight loss and metabolic benefits, but very high protein loads long term (over 6 months) may speed up a decline in your renal (kidney) function if you have kidney disease and increase your calcium loss in urine. This could predispose you to osteoporosis, kidney stones and other kidney problems. Scientists do not agree on the dangers of low carbohydrate diets and more longer term studies are needed.

Chapter 10
Carb quality: What you need to know about the glycemic index (GI)

While the amount of dietary carbohydrate is clearly a major determinant of the rise in blood glucose after eating, in practice, most people tend to eat much the same amount of carbohydrate from day to day and meal to meal. This makes the type of carbohydrate, particularly the glycemic index, or GI, of the carbohydrate food, an important consideration. Some foods, such as legumes and milk, naturally contain carbohydrates that are digested more slowly and have less impact on blood glucose. These foods are called low GI foods, and a low GI diet is one in which the meals are associated with lower blood glucose peaks after eating. On the other hand, a majority of modern starchy foods, including most breads and breakfast cereals, potatoes and rices, and even many processed wholegrain foods, are rapidly digested and absorbed and produce a high blood glucose peak or "glycemic spike." Sweets made with glucose, such as jelly beans and regular soft drinks, also have a relatively high GI. But surprisingly, many foods containing added sugars, such as ice cream, yogurt and chocolate, produce a relatively lower glucose response.

You can't guess the GI of a food by its appearance, ingredients or nutrient composition—it has to be tested in real human subjects who consume the food under highly standardized conditions. Professor David Jenkins and his colleagues at the University of Toronto developed and perfected the GI methodology, allowing us to classify all carbohydrate foods on a simple scale of 0 to 100 according to their glycemic impact. While the GI was considered controversial for some years, low GI diets are now recommended by major diabetes associations around the world. We now know the GI of about 2,500 different products, including most of the important carbohydrate sources in our diet. You can access a free searchable GI database at www.glycemicindex.com, as well as in the regularly updated *Shopper's Guide to GI Values*. You may also want to subscribe to the electronic *GI News* newsletter to read the most recent findings from around the world (http://ginews.blogspot.com/).

Using the GI is easy. You don't need to remember numbers or do any math. You simply swap your usual bread, breakfast cereal, rice or snack for a lower GI one (this for that). You just need to know which ones are low GI.

In 2009 scientists pooled results of nearly 30 years' research on the GI and its effect on people with diabetes and demonstrated that the use of the GI can lead to on average a 0.5 point decrease in HbA1c. This is equal to the effect that many diabetic medications and insulins have on blood glucose levels in people with diabetes. A drop in HbA1c of 0.5 points reduces the risk of diabetic complications by 10–20 percent—a highly significant reduction. Low GI diets also reduce the risk of having low blood sugar.

Here's what the GI can do for people with diabetes and prediabetes

We know from research that a diet based on low GI carbohydrate choices will:

- Reduce blood glucose "spikes"
- Improve markers of average blood glucose levels (that is, HbA1c)
- Improve insulin sensitivity
- Improve blood cholesterol levels, particularly LDL cholesterol
- Increase feelings of fullness after eating
- Reduce hunger between meals
- Increase the rate of weight loss (compared with a conventional diet)
- Reduce waist circumference (abdominal fat), and
- Help prevent weight regain over the longer term.

How do you know if a food has a low, medium or high GI?

To find the GI of your favorite brands you can:

- Check the nutritional label—some manufacturers now include GI
- Visit www.glycemicindex.com and search the free database
- Check the Shopper's Guide to GI Values (the edition is updated regularly), and/or
- Contact the manufacturer and ask (hound) them to have the food tested by an accredited lab.

What's glycemic load?

Your blood glucose level rises and falls when you eat a meal containing carbs. How high it rises and how long it stays high depends on the quality of the carbs (the GI) as well as the quantity. Glycemic load or GL combines both the quality and quantity of carbohydrate in one "number." It's the best way to compare blood glucose values of different types and amounts of food. The formula for calculating the GL of a particular food or meal is:

GL = (GI × the amount of carbohydrate) divided by 100.

Let's take a single apple as an example. It has a GI of 38, and it contains 13g of carbohydrate.

GL = 38 × 13/100 = 5

What about a small baked potato? Its GI is 85, and it contains 14g of carbohydrate.

GL = 85 × 14/100 = 12

So we can predict that our potato will have twice the glycemic effect of an apple. Think of GL as the amount of carbohydrate in a food "adjusted" for its glycemic potency.

Although the GL concept has been useful in scientific research, it's the GI that's been most helpful to people with diabetes. That's because a diet with a low GL, unfortunately, can be a "mixed bag," full of healthy low GI carbs in some cases, but low in carbs and full of the wrong sorts of fats (such as meat and butter) in others.

If you choose healthy low GI foods—at least one at each meal and monitor the amount of carbohydrate—chances are you'll be on the right track to blood glucose control.

Use the GI to identify your best carbohydrate choices, then take care with portion size to control the overall GL of your diet.

Chapter 11
How to change
the way you eat

"Get regular exercise." "Eat a healthy balanced diet." "Quit smoking."

"Easier said than done," you say.

Yes, it's much easier said than done. For most people with type 2 diabetes or prediabetes, managing what they eat and getting enough physical activity are the most challenging aspects of diabetes care because these really are lifestyle changes.

Limiting your food intake in the midst of plenty and getting more exercise in today's world are huge tasks on their own, let alone combined. That's why we've included a chapter that's devoted entirely to how to go about behavior changes when it comes to your eating habits. (And in Chapter 16, we cover ideas for activating your day.)

Your current food habits are the product of many factors: your cultural and family background, childhood experiences, personal tastes, family preferences, budget, the season, food availability, appetite, mood. And that's just to name a few. That's why changing what you eat is more than simply putting something else on your plate. Changing what you eat can challenge your beliefs, relationships and resourcefulness.

Although you have to make the decision to change, you'll most likely benefit from some outside help and support. That's why we suggest that everyone with diabetes see a qualified dietitian. As you saw in Chapter 5, when we ran through what's involved in a diabetes management plan, it recommended you see a dietitian when you are first diagnosed and have routine follow-up. Because you are looking at managing a life-long condition, it makes sense to find someone you are comfortable seeing regularly. A good place to start is to ask your doctor for a recommendation.

When **you have diabetes, you have it for the rest of your life**, but the health complications, such as blindness, kidney failure or heart disease, take years to develop, so it can be hard to focus on the changes that you need to make here and now.

Tried and true tips for changing eating and activity habits

- **Aim to make changes gradually.**
- **Acknowledge your stage of change.**
  People don't make changes instantaneously; they work up to them. For some, the first step is increasing awareness of their eating habits by keeping a food diary. This can really help you identify obstacles such as lack of time, traveling, socializing or working late. Once you have identified the obstacles, you can do something about them.
- **Try the easiest changes first.**
  Start with something easy that is realistic and that's achievable. There's not much point aiming to eat fresh fish three times a week if it's not readily available where you live. Nothing inspires like success, so start with changing a habit that will give you confidence to go on. A track record of small successes will give you the momentum you need for the challenges ahead.

- **Break big changes into a number of smaller ones.**

  Don't try to change everything at once. Trying to quit smoking and drinking, start eating better, and exercising all at the same time could leave you feeling discouraged and ready to give up. Break the change down from a large behavior (quit smoking) into smaller ones (not buying cigarettes, smoking fewer and fewer each day, eliminating the after dinner cigarette, etc.).

- **Accept lapses in your habits: it's part of being human.**

  Don't expect 100 percent success. Giving up comfort foods can cause depression and resentment, so factor in a little treat every now and then. And don't be too hard on yourself when you can't resist that piece of cheesecake. Lapses are a natural part of developing new habits. Falling over is easy, but getting up, dusting yourself off and keeping on takes real effort. Watch toddlers learning to walk and take a leaf out of their book.

Helping yourself toward healthier eating habits

Become aware of non-hungry eating

Food is part of socializing, celebrating and comforting, and eating gives us something to do when we are bored. We eat food for a whole range of reasons which have nothing to do with hunger. We eat:

- So as not to offend a host
- Because we feel anxious or depressed
- To finish off what the kids have left
- Just because it looks good, or because it's there, and
- Because we feel we have to leave nothing on our plate.

  Non-hungry eating isn't wrong, but it can contribute to overeating, and you need to be aware of it if you are going to do anything about it. Try to identify what triggers you to eat when you're not particularly hungry, and work on eliminating or reducing those triggers. If an argument with your partner sends you to the cookie jar, deliberately do something else—taking a walk, for instance—to work out the emotion instead of suppressing it with food.

Think about what to eat, rather than what not to eat

What happens if someone asks you not to think about a pink elephant? You imagine it, right? The future is what we imagine. So rather than thinking of what you don't want to eat, think of what you do. If you crave chocolate, have some, but buy only one tiny bar of your favorite and relish it.

Planning the meals you are going to eat reduces the likelihood that you'll go off track. Plan the week's main meals and shop once for the ingredients you'll need. Make a shopping list of healthy foods, including some favorites that you always buy. Two of our favorites are nut bars, and fruit and muesli bread. The bread is a satisfying snack anytime at home, and the bars are great for food on the go.

Eat regularly

Have you ever noticed that the hungrier you are, the more tempting high calorie foods like chocolate, cookies and chips are? And the harder it is to stop at one? You'll find it easier to eat normally if you learn to graze on low GI carbs.

Make overeating as hard as you can

When you go to have a slice of bread, take out one slice, then seal up the bag and put the loaf away. Put the spreads and toppings away before you sit down to eat. Out of sight generally means out of mind. Keep those occasional foods out of sight—better still, don't buy them routinely.

If it's healthy, keep it handy

In your face and ready to eat! Keep washed, shiny apples or crunchy snow peas in an attractive bowl in the fridge; dried fruit in a jar on your desk; packaged instant salads for convenience; pre-sliced tomato and cucumber in the fridge, ready to use on sandwiches. These are just a few of the ways you can increase your chances of eating the types of foods you planned to eat.

Minimize distractions while you're eating

If you're sitting in front of the TV with a bag of chips or a bar of chocolate, it is very easy to absent-mindedly down it all. Focus on and savor what you are eating.

Get support from others

Whether it's from your family, friends, work colleagues or health professionals, get as much help as you can. Find a buddy who also wants to get into shape. When your motivation dips, theirs will pull you along. If someone seems to be sabotaging your efforts, let them know how they could help. For example, they could agree to change to low GI bread. There are things you may need to negotiate. Be prepared to lead by example, and to ignore the hecklers . . . and you may convince others you are onto something good.

Cope with stress (without using food)

Stress can take many forms. It can appear emotionally as anxiety, worry or depression. Or you can experience it physically, as pain or illness. Situations such as a confrontation with another person or a near-miss accident can trigger the so-called fight or flight response, which is associated with the release of stress hormones.

For people with diabetes, stress often results in elevated blood glucose levels because these stress hormones trigger the release of stored glucose. This energy-mobilizing effect helps people who don't have diabetes deal better with their environment, but it is no help for people with diabetes. They find it harder to regain normal glucose equilibrium. This can lead to chronic high blood glucose.

If you have diabetes, try to find ways to manage your stress without resorting to the cookie jar, alcohol or cigarettes. Here's a list of some of the things that may help you manage stress better:

- **Self-knowledge**. Get to know your body's normal reactions so that you can recognize when you are tense. Shallow breathing and a fast pulse are often an indication of your body's reaction to stress
- **Relax**. Deep breathing is a natural relaxant. Try to take several deep breaths each hour
- **Talk**. Talking to other people can be a valuable way to deal with your problems and reduce the stress associated with them
- **Walk**. Physical activity will help you reduce tension and can be a great way to clear your mind
- **Smile and laugh**. It's therapeutic, so take any opportunity you can to do it
- **Make lists**. This will help you sort out your priorities and give you a feeling of control over what you want to do. Make a list of 10 things that make you happy—a good coffee? A good book? A hot bath? Make sure you indulge occasionally
- **Have fun**. Learn to play a little. Keep up your hobbies and try to get out of the house regularly, even if it's only for short outings
- **Explore**. New activities may help you relax such as massage, listening to music, meditating and yoga
- **Believe**. Your religious or spiritual beliefs could be very supportive and help you to see a way forward, and

- **Be aware of your needs**. Give priority to meeting them when you can. Take time to rest when you are tired, to eat when you're hungry. Be kind to yourself.

If none of these solutions seems to help, it's a good idea to see a trained counselor. Behavioral stress management programs do work.

Chapter 12
Planning healthy meals using a plate model

A basic main meal, whether it's traditional foods or foods with a Mediterranean or Asian twist, consists of some sort of meat with vegetables and potato, or rice, pasta or noodles. There's nothing wrong with this as a starting point; a little finetuning of the proportions to match the plate model will ensure a healthy, balanced meal.

What is the plate model? We didn't create it, but we use it and recommend it because it is simple and it works. It's an easy-to-learn aid to visualizing what to put on your plate. It is adaptable to different cuisines and handy to take to restaurants. You can use it for any sized servings as long as you keep the food to the proportions shown.

You can use the plate model alongside other dietary tools you find helpful, such as the daily food guide or carbohydrate counting (see Chapter 9). And as long as you choose foods that fit into the key recommendations— upping the good fats, cutting back on saturated fat and being choosy about your carbs—you're on track to a healthy diet for managing your diabetes and losing weight (if you need to).

In our experience, there are some situations where people find the plate model particularly useful. They are:

- When you have just found out you have diabetes and you feel overwhelmed by all the dietary changes you need to make
- When you want a simple diet plan to follow
- When you are having a hard time understanding other diet methods, such as using a food guide for diabetes (similar to the food guide pyramid), counting carbohydrates in your diet, or using lists that group foods according to nutrient content (diabetic exchange lists)
- If you have difficulty reading
- If you learn best by visualizing, and
- When you are eating away from home.

If you are already using other methods, the plate model might be another dietary tool to help you plan interesting, well-balanced meals, especially when you are trying out new recipes or a different cuisine.

With Asian meals, where food is typically served in individual bowls, the same principle applies—imagine three bowls: a small bowl each for the rice or noodles and for the protein part of the meal and a large bowl for the vegetables.

With the plate model there are just three simple steps to a healthy meal.

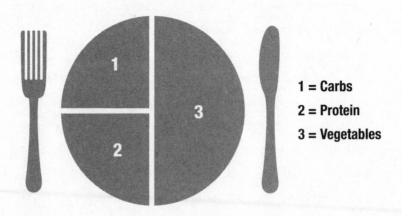

1 = Carbs
2 = Protein
3 = Vegetables

On the plate

1. Carbohydrate-rich foods

How much? One-quarter of the plate

What? Bread and cereals (choose low GI types) and other starchy foods such as potatoes, sweet potatoes, yams, taro, legumes, sweet corn, pasta, noodles and rice

2. Protein-rich foods

How much? One-quarter of the plate

What? Meat, chicken, fish, eggs, tofu and alternatives such as legumes, milk or yogurt

3. Vegetables

How much? Half the plate

What? Brighten your plate with a variety of colorful vegetables. Try leafy green and salad vegetables, green beans and peas, broccoli and cauliflower, zucchini and baby squash, onions and leeks, fennel and asparagus, for starters. Think of vegetables as free foods that are full of fiber and essential nutrients, and that fill you up without adding extra calories.

Note: When it comes to vegetables, potato, sweet corn, sweet potato, yams, taro and legumes count as carbohydrate foods.

Outside the plate

Fruit and/or milk products as a beverage or dessert on occasion.

For a more detailed guide to putting together meals over the day, use the daily food guides that we have included throughout Part 3.

Chapter 13
Snacks—Why? What? What not?

There are some who overdo it, some who don't want to do it at all, and some who aren't aware that they are doing it. What? Snacking—taking a bite to eat between meals, morning coffee, refreshments, nibbles.

Diet sheets for people with diabetes often include a recommendation to eat little and often, including between-meal snacks. This can cause a lot of concern.

If you take some types of insulin or pills, you may need to eat some form of carbohydrate between meals to stop your blood glucose dropping too low—newer forms of medication make it less likely that you will need to do this. Besides preventing low blood sugar, this chapter looks at some of the reasoning behind eating more than three times a day.

Why snack?

Even if you're not taking any diabetes medication, lots of people with diabetes or prediabetes want to know whether it's better to eat many small meals rather than less frequent large meals.

There's no doubt that snacks can make a significant contribution to a healthy diet, and for little children in particular, they're recommended—

it's harder for them to get sufficient calories. Even for adults, regular snacks can prevent extreme hunger and may reduce the amount of food eaten at meals, which can be helpful for blood glucose levels.

Studies examining the metabolic effects of small, frequent meals ("grazing") versus two or three large meals have found that blood glucose and blood fat levels may improve when meal frequency increases. There's also some evidence that you will reap metabolic benefits by eating at set times rather than at different times on different days.

This doesn't mean you should be eating more food.

It means spreading the same amount of food over more frequent and smaller meals. It seems that if you spread the nutrient load more evenly over the day, you reduce the load on the beta cells and maximize insulin sensitivity. Researchers have seen this effect in people without diabetes, too. Although it has not yet been proven in controlled trials, it may also be that small, frequent meals lower the risk of developing diabetes by reducing the periodic "surges" in insulin that follow large meals.

There's also evidence that eating foods with carbohydrate in them at regular intervals can improve your mood and your mental performance. A steady supply of glucose from snacks has been shown to improve short-term memory and has been linked to better attention and number recall.

What happens if you're a non-snacker and you don't feel hungry between meals? Although you may be able to last for several hours without eating because you are busy or preoccupied, going a long time between meals generally means you will be hungrier when you do eat and therefore driven to more energy-dense (more calories per bite) foods.

The jury is still out on whether or not snacking is good for your weight. There are pros and cons. There is circumstantial evidence that eating three meals a day may help you manage your weight. The French, for example, generally eat only three meals a day, with little or no snacking between, whereas we tend to eat small quantities of food fairly often. However, there's another big difference in eating habits between the French and the Americans that may be even more important: in France, meals are more often prepared and eaten in the home, not from fast food restaurants or packaged meals.

It is possible that healthy snacking on lower fat, higher carbohydrate, low GI high fiber foods will stave off your "hunger pangs" and help you stick to moderate servings at meal times. Grazing can be a healthy way to live and still maintain or lose weight—but it depends on what you eat and how much you eat. Very physically active people should probably graze on higher carbohydrate snacks to make sure a continual supply of glucose is available to their hard-working muscles.

However, snacking is definitely bad news for your teeth. Each time you eat, the bacteria in plaque attack your tooth enamel. For your dental health, you need to leave a minimum of 2 hours between drinks or snacks.

Slowly sipping sweetened or acidic drinks (and this includes "diet" soft drinks) also has harmful effects on your teeth because it causes "dental erosion" (loss of tooth enamel caused by acid attack). It's better for your teeth to drink relatively quickly, and give your teeth a period of at least 2 hours for "rest and recovery."

In the end, it is your overall food intake that counts with weight matters, not whether you only eat breakfast, lunch and dinner or graze throughout the day.

Snacking: the bottom line

People who snack and eat regularly:

- Have a reduced risk of low blood glucose levels (hypoglycemia)
- Show improved insulin sensitivity with lower postprandial (after-eating) insulin levels

- May have lower blood cholesterol levels
- Perform better in memory and problem-solving tasks, and
- May be less likely to overeat at meals.

What to snack on

What to choose for snacks can be a real challenge given the huge (and tempting) range of individually packaged bars, cookies, chips, dairy desserts, muffins and drinks on the market, most of which have eye-catching packaging that tells you they have some vital nutritional benefit.

In reality, the best snack foods don't usually come in packaging at all—but it may boost their sales if it did. The best snacks are portable, inexpensive, nutritionally faultless foods. What are they? Fresh fruit, of course. An apple, a banana, a bunch of grapes, a pear or a nectarine or a mandarin or orange.

Think ahead

It is a good idea to plan between-meal snacks ahead of time. If you leave your snacks to chance, you probably won't make the best choice when you walk in the door at the end of the day, ravenous. Dinner won't be ready for at least another hour, so what do you do? Well, it depends:

- If you've kept some nutritious snacks in your workplace, car or bag, you could have taken the edge off your appetite with something healthy on the way home
- You might have prepared a plate of chopped fruit, carrot and celery sticks with hummus in the morning and tossed it into the fridge, or
- You might have bought some lower fat yogurt, crackers and reduced fat cheese or roasted unsalted nuts and seeds.

Sweet treats with a low glycemic impact

Allow yourself small indulgences. It's OK to give yourself a sweet treat a couple of times a week, but don't eat a king-size Mars bar every day to satisfy a craving for chocolate. Go for a smaller sized chocolate—and resist those cravings as often as you can. One of the things that makes treat foods a treat is keeping them as occasional eating.

What not to snack on

Have you ever sat in front of the TV with a bag of chips or nuts, thinking you'll eat just a few, and before you know it you're licking the salt off your fingers and wondering where they've all gone? The problem with snacking is control. That's one reason why it can be one of the worst dietary habits.

It's the way we snack that can be the problem—what we choose, when we have it and why we're eating it. Beware of triggers that lead you to snack on something you hadn't planned on. The TV ad late at night (or at the movies) for some delectably creamy ice cream; the bag of chips that jumps into your hands from a vending machine as you are walking by; the chocolate bars that gleam and smile at you when you stop to buy gas.

Risky snacking scenarios to avoid

- Replacing meals with snacks because you don't have the time or the food preparation skills, or you're feeling lazy and unmotivated
- At football or other sports events
- At the movies
- Watching TV
- When you're upset—emotional non-hungry eating, and
- Eating when you're away from home, such as when you're out shopping.

Q&A

Is it true that people with diabetes should eat between-meal snacks and supper before going to bed?

Children and adults with type 1 diabetes often need to have between-meal snacks and supper to prevent low blood sugar. A small supper of low GI carbohydrate before bed can reduce the risk of nocturnal hypoglycemia in people with type 1 diabetes, although pump technology and new insulins are making this less necessary.

People with prediabetes or type 2 diabetes who aren't using insulin probably don't need to snack to help with blood glucose control, though there may be exceptions.

In today's calorie-dense environment there is mounting evidence that poorly chosen between-meal snacks lead to weight gain, which may in turn make your diabetes worse.

You should aim to have three moderate size meals based around low GI carbohydrates to keep your blood glucose levels stable throughout the day. If you find you are going low between main meals, ask your diabetes team to review your blood glucose-lowering medications.

Chapter 14
Renovate your recipes

Managing diabetes doesn't mean you have to throw out your favorite cookbooks and head to the local bookstore for new ones. Many recipes can easily be adapted to suit healthy eating guidelines. In this chapter we set out four key strategies to use when modifying recipes and four sample recipe make-overs to inspire you to put on an apron, pick up a wooden spoon and take charge in the kitchen!

A note of caution: modifying recipes can involve a certain amount of trial and error. And it certainly helps if you have some cooking experience and an idea of what's likely to work and what definitely won't (read: be prepared for some flops). But you'll reap the reward when your health—and your family—thank you for a super-healthy, super-delicious "re-creation." And you can have a lot of fun in the kitchen experimenting.

With diabetes, the general aims in modifying a recipe are to:

- Reduce the amount and improve the quality of the fat
- Lower the GI
- Boost the fiber content, and
- Reduce the salt content.

So how do you go about it? There are four basic strategies you can use. You may need to use one or all four, depending on the recipe:

1. *Substitute* healthier versions of ingredients: replace full fat milk with lower fat milk, for instance.

2. *Add* lower calorie ingredients to make a higher calorie dish go further: use vegetables as part of the filling in a quiche, for example.

3. *Eliminate* the ingredient you're trying to avoid: leave the cream out, for example.

4. *Reduce* the amount of the ingredient you're trying to cut back on: use one slice of bacon instead of two, for example.

Fat—how to reduce the amount and improve the quality

Delectable ingredients such as butter, cream, bacon, cheese and chocolate need to stay on the supermarket shelf and out of your shopping cart if you're going to create anything approaching a diabetes-friendly recipe.

Substitute

- Olive oil for butter when sautéing
- Lemon juice and black pepper as a dressing for steamed vegetables rather than melted butter
- Canola oil for butter or margarine when baking
- Avocado, hummus or fat-reduced margarine on a sandwich instead of butter
- Low-fat evaporated milk, buttermilk, lower fat natural yogurt or reduced fat or skim milk thickened with cornstarch in place of cream for savory sauces
- Reduced fat cheese (even partially) for regular full fat cheeses (NB: most mozzarella is lower in fat than many other cheeses), and
- 2–3 sheets of filo pastry brushed with milk or a little olive oil for regular puff or shortcrust pastry.

Add

- Slivered nuts, sunflower seeds or pumpkin seeds instead of bacon bits to salads

- Avocado instead of cheese or margarine to a sandwich
- Lower fat natural yogurt instead of sour cream to a salad dressing, and
- A handful of nuts to stir-fries or in baked goods such as muffins and cakes.

Eliminate

- Fat from meat before cooking by trimming it away, and removing the skin from chicken pieces
- Fat from soups and stews by cooking ahead, chilling and then skimming the fat from the top, and
- Fat from cooking by using pan liners when frying, and using low-fat cooking methods such as steaming, grilling or microwaving.

Reduce

- The amount of oil when stir-frying by adding a splash of water or stock (don't add them at the same time!)
- The amount of cheese by using half the amount of a sharper flavored type like parmesan, or by replacing slices of block cheese with a sprinkle of reduced fat grated cheese
- The amount of oil used when roasting vegetables by partially cooking them in the microwave first and then spraying or brushing them with oil and baking until crisp
- Saturated fat by using reduced fat sour cream, lower fat yogurt, buttermilk or reduced fat ricotta cheese as an alternative to full fat sour cream
- Baked cheesy toppings by using half the cheese, mixed with traditional rolled or stoneground oats, breadcrumbs or wheatgerm, and
- Margarine or butter in cakes by experimenting with fruit puree or egg whites as a partial substitute.

Keep fat in perspective

Sometimes you can't replace a high fat ingredient or switch to a lower fat cooking method without compromising the end product. Not all the food you eat has to be low-fat. The key is balance. As well as modifying some of your existing recipes, you can also find new recipes that are similar to your recipes but have less fat or higher quality fat and more nutritious ingredients.

And remember, there's another way to control your fat intake. Reduce the amount of food you normally consume and fill up with vegetables instead.

GI—how to reduce the glycemic impact and lower the glycemic load

Substitute

- Unprocessed oat bran (as a partial substitute) for flour in baked muffins and cakes
- Low GI alternatives such as sweet corn, lentils or cannellini bean mash for high GI foods such as regular mashed potato
- A pure wildflower honey or maple syrup or agave nectar for sugar as a sweetener
- Sourdough or low GI bread for regular bread
- Soy flour or chickpea flour as a lower GI alternative to wholemeal flour if making flatbreads, and
- Basmati or low GI brown rice for regular rice.

Eliminate

- Fluffy high GI white breads: go for dense wholegrain or authentic sourdough instead
- Large servings of high GI foods and ingredients, including most potatoes and floury products, and
- Light crispy crackers and packaged snacks: eat fruit or a low-fat dairy product instead.

Add

- Something acidic to the meal or dish, such as vinaigrette over salad, lemon juice over vegetables, yogurt or buttermilk in baked goods
- Dried fruit or fresh diced apple or pear to a muffin mix
- Natural lower fat yogurt to a curry and rice meal
- A low GI food to a high GI food to give you something in between
- Legumes to meals: bean mix to a salad, lentils, chickpeas to a casserole, for instance, and
- Alternative sweeteners instead of sugar—see Chapter 15.

Reduce

- The amount of sugar added to recipes: look at the overall quantity of sugar in relation to how many servings (½ cup of sugar in a recipe that serves 10 people will have very little effect on your blood glucose levels, for example)
- Your serving size of rice- or pasta-based meals (add extra vegetables to fill the gap), and
- Snacks of cookies, crackers, muffins, scones, doughnuts, cakes, high GI white bread and rolls: replace them with fruit, low-fat yogurt, nuts and vegetable sticks.

Fiber—how to boost

Substitute

- A mixture of wholemeal and white flour or add a little bran: you may need to add a little extra liquid to keep the recipe moist
- Wholegrain bread, wholegrain breadcrumbs, grainy muffins, wholemeal flatbread, wholemeal rolls, authentic sourdough bread wherever you've previously used plain white, and
- Dried fruit for sweet treats.

Eliminate

- Low fiber high GI cereals from your breakfast shelf.

Add

- Extra vegetables to casseroles, soups and sauces
- Leave the skin on fruits and vegetables (such as apples or potatoes) when using them in recipes.
- Fresh or dried fruit in bread and cookie recipes
- Legumes (beans, chickpeas and lentils, home-cooked or canned) to meals
- A small amount of processed wheat bran cereal to meatloaf or even a breakfast smoothie, and
- Sautéed mushrooms, other vegetables or some lentils in a spaghetti sauce.

Reduce

- The number of times you buy high GI white bread, white bread rolls, English muffins, muffins and pancakes, which are usually low fiber forms of these foods.

Salt—how to reduce the amount you eat

Substitute

- A salt substitute (such as potassium chloride) in cooking
- "Salt reduced" or "no added salt" varieties for regular canned foods, and
- Spices such as freshly ground black pepper, chili powder, paprika, mustard and cardamom for salt.

Eliminate

- Salt from the dining table
- Sea salt, rock salt, vegetable salt, celery salt, garlic salt, chicken salt: they are not suitable substitutes for salt.

Add

- Other flavorings, such as fresh herbs (try parsley, basil, oregano, chives, rosemary, coriander, mint, sage, thyme, tarragon and marjoram), and
- Lemon juice, onions, ginger, shallots, vinegar, wine as flavorings.

Reduce

- Your intake of foods high in added sodium
- Canned and packaged soups
- Canned vegetables
- Bottled sauces, including tomato, BBQ, worcestershire, soy and fish sauce
- Stock cubes and powders
- Salty snack foods such as chips, pretzels, roasted nuts or savory crackers
- Olives and pickles
- Deli meats, bacon and other cured meats
- Cheeses, and
- Restaurant and fast foods.

Chapter 15
Sugar and sweeteners: The real deal

Do you feel guilty every time you enjoy something sweet? Do you think diabetes equals no sugar? Join the club. Many people think that if something tastes good, it must be bad for them. And many people with diabetes, and even their doctors, mistakenly believe that sugar consumption is the most important explanation for high blood glucose readings.

While we now know that's not the case, old habits die hard. Traditionally, people with diabetes have been told to replace all sugar with an artificial sweetener and to drink diet soft drinks. It's enough to make some people with diabetes turn their backs on all dietary advice.

But wanting something sweet is instinctive, and hard to ignore. It is part of our "hardwiring." In our hunter-gatherer past, fruits, berries and honey were our only source of carbohydrate energy. Starch was hard to come by.

You'll be relieved to know that most diabetes organizations all around the world no longer advise strict avoidance of refined sugar or sugary foods. This is one of the happy spin-offs from research on the GI—recognition that both sugary foods and starchy foods raise your blood glucose.

Furthermore, dozens of studies indicate that moderate amounts of added sugar in diabetic diets (for example 30–50 grams per day) does not result in either poor control or weight gain. Yes, a soft drink can be a concentrated source of calories, but so can a fruit juice or an alcoholic drink.

You can enjoy refined or "added" sugar in moderation—that's about 30–50 grams (6–10 teaspoons) a day—an amount that most people consume without trying hard. Try to include sweetened foods that provide more than just calories—dairy foods, breakfast cereals, oatmeal with brown sugar, jam on wholegrain toast, etc. Even the World Health Organization says "a moderate intake of sugar-rich foods can provide for a palatable and nutritious diet." So forget the guilt trip and allow yourself the pleasure of sweetness.

Should we be concerned about fructose?

One form of sugar, fructose or fruit sugar, has been hitting the headlines because of the alarmist view that it is "toxic" to our metabolism and should be consumed in minimal amounts. We don't agree and neither do the experts! Indeed, we believe that avoiding fructose could do more harm than good.

Fructose represents about half the natural sugars in fruit and vegetables. It is also one half of the sucrose molecule (that's the one in cane or refined sugar) and as much as 70 percent of the total sugars in honey. Fructose has a low GI (equivalent to 20) and in normal quantities it contributes to better diabetes control and lower blood pressure.

In the United States, average fructose consumption from all sources is 62 grams a day (12½ teaspoons) with even the highest consumers eating 90 grams (18 teaspoons). Nutritional analysis of a typical low GI menu generates 70 grams of sugar per day, of which 25–30 grams would be fructose.

Can fructose contribute to weight gain?

Of course! Like all carbohydrates, it contains 4 calories per gram, yet that's a lot less than the calories in a gram of fat (9 calories per gram) or alcohol (7 calories per gram). Recent expert reviews of all available human research on fructose concluded that fructose does not cause weight gain when it is substituted for other carbohydrates in diets providing similar calories. Consuming added fructose *at very high doses* (more than 100 grams or 20 teaspoons per day) may modestly increase body weight, but this effect is most likely due to the extra calories rather than the fructose.

From an evolutionary perspective, fructose was an important component of intelligent primate diets. Our human ancestors adored sweet berries and honey and made sweet drinks using both honey and floral nectars. In the 1980s, we analyzed hundreds of traditional Aboriginal bushfoods, including sugarbag (bush honey) and dried bush fruits, such as the bush tomato *Solanum central*, which is 80 percent (by weight) sugar. In other parts of the world, apiculture, the art of raising bees, was widely practiced, even by the poor. Indeed at certain times in history, consumption of honey may well have rivaled our current consumption of refined sugar.

Strict avoidance of sugars and fructose reduces the enjoyment and quality of life for millions of people who enjoy a "spoonful of sugar." The take-home message is that a moderate consumption of fructose is compatible with a palatable and nutritious diet.

What about alternative sweeteners?

Alternatives to sugar are widely used by people with diabetes to sweeten drinks (tea and coffee) and foods (breakfast cereals); to sweeten recipes (for cakes and desserts); and in low calorie commercial products (soft drinks, fruit punch, jams, gelatins and yogurts).

They do give you sweetness with fewer calories, and usually with less effect on blood glucose levels, but there are differences among them.

Not all alternative sweeteners are the same—some have just as many calories as sugar, but others have no calories at all; some are thousands (yes thousands) of times sweeter than sugar; others are not very sweet at all. One thing they all have in common, however, is that they are more expensive than sugar.

There are lots of brands of sweeteners on the supermarket shelves, but essentially there are two main types:

- Nutritive sweeteners, and
- Non-nutritive sweeteners.

What's the difference?

Nutritive sweeteners

Nutritive sweeteners are simply those that provide some calories and, as the name suggests, nutrients. Sugar, for example, is a nutritive sweetener, but so are things like sorbitol and maltodextrin. They have differing effects on blood glucose levels.

Old-fashioned table sugar stands up well under scrutiny—it is the second sweetest after fructose, has only a moderate GI, is the best value for money and is the easiest to use in cooking. And because it generally has a lower GI than the refined flour used in baking, it can actually lower the GI of many recipes! Less refined sweeteners like raw sugar, honey, golden syrup and pure (100 percent) maple syrup also provide small amounts of calcium, potassium and magnesium.

The sugar alcohols, such as sorbitol, mannitol and maltitol, are generally not as sweet as table sugar, provide fewer calories and have less of an impact on blood glucose levels. To overcome their lack of sweetness, food manufacturers usually combine them with non-nutritive sweeteners to help keep the calorie count down and minimize the effect on blood glucose levels. This will be shown in the ingredients list on the food label.

The nutritive sweeteners such as sorbitol, mannitol, xylitol and maltitol, and maltitol syrup, may have a laxative effect or cause gas or diarrhea if you consume them in large amounts. Foods that contain more than 10 grams per 100 grams of these alternative sweeteners, or more than 25 grams per 100 grams of sorbitol, isomalt, or polydextrose, carry warning statements on their labels about the possible laxative effect. These products can be a particular problem for children and adolescents because of their smaller body size.

Used in sensible quantities, fructose certainly rivals table sugar as a good all-round sweetener. It stands out from the crowd, being nearly twice as sweet as sugar, providing the same number of calories, but having only one-third the GI, so you can use less fructose to achieve the same level of sweetness and as a result consume fewer calories and experience a much smaller rise in your blood glucose levels. Its main drawback is cost.

If you have read alarmist reports about fructose and blood fats and/or insulin resistance, remember that most of this research was on rats and mice fed excessive quantities of pure added fructose—more than someone with even the sweetest tooth could tolerate. There is no evidence that fructose has adverse effects in people with diabetes consuming normal quantities (e.g., less than 100 grams of added fructose per day). Average added fructose consumption is 41 grams per day in the United States. Even then, most of it comes from added high fructose corn syrup, which is half fructose and half glucose.

Non-nutritive sweeteners

Non-nutritive sweeteners (such as Equal, Splenda or saccharin) are all much sweeter than table sugar and essentially have no effect on your blood glucose levels because most are used in such small quantities and are either not absorbed into or metabolized by the body. Because they are only used in minute amounts, the number of calories they provide is insignificant.

What's best to use for cooking?

The non-nutritive sweeteners that are made of protein molecules often break down when heated at high temperatures for long periods, thus losing their sweetness. For this reason, they are not always ideal for baking. The best non-nutritive sweeteners to cook with are Splenda and saccharin and, to a lesser extent, Equal Spoonful.

Are they safe?

As a group, non-nutritive sweeteners have been studied more thoroughly than any other type of food additive. Questions about the safety of saccharin were raised when it was first discovered over 135 years ago, and its effect on human health has been monitored ever since. The same is true of more recent sweeteners such as aspartame and sucralose. There is no convincing evidence so far that any of the non-nutritive sweeteners on the market have any negative effects on our health.

While the non-nutritive sweeteners available in North America are considered safe for everyone, some health professionals opt for caution and recommend that pregnant women avoid saccharin. This is because it crosses the placenta to the growing fetus and can also be found in breast milk.

Also, studies in rats have shown an increased risk of bladder cancer due to saccharin use. To put this in perspective, remember that saccharin was used widely after World War II because there was a worldwide sugar shortage, and we did not see an increase in bladder cancer over that period. So it seems unlikely that the sweetener is a problem for pregnant women or those who are breastfeeding. However, some women still choose to avoid this non-nutritive sweetener.

What about stevia and monk fruit?

Stevia has become popular with people seeking a more "natural" alternative sweetener. Its natural reputation stems from the fact that it is derived from a sweet-tasting herb (*Stevia rebaudiana*), although stevia sweetener comes from a highly purified part of the plant (steviol glycosides). The leaves of the herb can be used as a sweetener themselves, and in the dried form less than 2 tablespoons of crushed leaves can replace the sweetness of about 1 cup of sugar. In commercial powdered products the steviol glycosides are usually combined with other substances to provide bulk or improve taste and texture. You can buy stevia in purified liquid and powder form and also in combination with other sugar replacers in tablet, powdered and granulated form.

Like stevia, monk fruit (*luo han guo*), from Central Asia, is another natural alternative sweetener. The sweet extract of monk fruit, which is 200–400x sweeter than sugar, is usually combined with a dextrin or the sugar alcohol, erythritol, in commercial granulated products.

Both stevia and monk fruit sweetener are suitable for cooking. Both are virtually calorie free, tooth-friendly and have no impact on blood glucose levels.

Phenylketonuria and aspartame

Food and beverages in North America that contain aspartame must carry a warning for people with phenylketonuria. Phenylketonuria is a rare genetic disease, which is characterized by an inability of the body to utilize the essential amino acid, phenylalanine. About 1 in 10,000 newborn babies is affected with the condition. Managing this disease includes sticking to a low protein diet with particular emphasis on avoiding foods high in phenylalanine. As aspartame contains a significant amount of phenylalanine, it is not recommended for people with phenylketonuria.

What should you do?

Replacing table sugar with alternative sweeteners may have some health benefits but these come at a cost. To achieve the best of both worlds we suggest that you use your favourite alternative sweetener in those dishes that normally require a significant amount of added sugar (half a cup or more). For the rest of the time, just have a teaspoon or two of sugar and enjoy it.

Authorities such as the American Diabetes Association always recommend that people use a variety of sweeteners, including aspartame, sucralose, acesulphame K and saccharin so that the likelihood of excessive consumption of any one sweetener is reduced.

Blends: The best of both worlds?

Splenda Sugar Blend for Baking is a blend of ordinary table sugar and sucralose, a non-nutritive sweetener. By adding sucralose to sugar, you get the best of both worlds: an intense sweetener with ferwer calories, but the cooking properties of sugar. Its only downside is its cost—nearly three times that of table sugar.

Nutritive sweeteners

Fructose GI 19 4 calories per gram 11 calories per teaspoon table sugar equivalent*	Fructose or fruit sugar has a relatively small effect on blood glucose levels. It is nearly twice as sweet as table sugar, but it has the same number of calories per gram. Sweetness relative to table sugar = up to 70% more depending on the temperature of the food
Glucose GI 100 4 calories per gram 26 calories per teaspoon table sugar equivalent*	Glucose is the sugar found in blood. When eaten, it causes blood glucose levels to rise rapidly. It is not as sweet as table sugar, but it has the same number of calories. Sweetness relative to table sugar = 25% less
Golden syrup GI 63 3 calories per gram 11 calories per teaspoon table sugar equivalent*	Golden syrup has a moderate effect on blood glucose levels, very similar to table sugar. It is sweeter than table sugar, and it has fewer calories per gram. Sweetness relative to table sugar = 33% more
Grape syrup GI 52 4 calories per gram 16 calories per teaspoon table sugar equivalent*	Grape syrup or nectar has a moderate effect on blood glucose levels. It is a little sweeter than table sugar, but it has the same number of calories. Sweetness relative to table sugar = 20% more

Honey
GI range 35–64

4 calories per gram

20 calories per teaspoon table sugar equivalent*

Honey has a moderate effect on blood glucose levels depending on whether it is a blend or a pure floral honey. The pure floral honeys appear to have lower GIs. On average, honey is slightly less sweet than table sugar, but it has the same number of calories.
Sweetness relative to table sugar = about the same

Isomalt
GI 60

3 calories per gram

26 calories per teaspoon table sugar equivalent*

Isomalt is very poorly absorbed, so it has essentially no effect on blood glucose levels when consumed in typical amounts. It is only half as sweet as table sugar, but it has fewer calories and may have a laxative effect if eaten in large quantities.
Sweetness relative to table sugar = half as sweet

Lactose
GI 46

4 calories per gram

120 calories per teaspoon table sugar equivalent*

Lactose is the sugar found in milk. When eaten, it causes blood glucose levels to rise slowly. It is not very sweet at all, but it has the same number of calories as table sugar.
Sweetness relative to table sugar = 85% less sweet

Maltitol

GI 69

3 calories per gram

21 calories per teaspoon table sugar equivalent*

Maltitol is poorly absorbed, so it has little effect on blood glucose levels when consumed in typical amounts. It is only three-quarters as sweet as table sugar and has the same number of calories. It may have a laxative effect and cause gas and diarrhea if eaten in large quantities.
Sweetness relative to table sugar = 25% less sweet

Maltodextrins

GI not known

4 calories per gram

35 calories per teaspoon table sugar equivalent*

Maltodextrins are short chain glucose polymers with a GI similar to that of glucose. They are only half as sweet as table sugar and have the same number of calories.
Sweetness relative to table sugar = half as sweet

Maltose

GI 105

4 calories per gram

60 calories per teaspoon table sugar equivalent*

Maltose or malt causes blood glucose levels to rise rapidly. It is only one-third as sweet as table sugar and has the same number of calories.
Sweetness relative to table sugar = 67% less sweet

Mannitol

GI n/a

2 calories per gram

15 calories per teaspoon table sugar equivalent*

Mannitol has no effect on blood glucose levels. It is only three-quarters as sweet as table sugar, but it has only half the number of calories. It may have a laxative effect and cause gas and diarrhea if eaten in large quantities.
Sweetness relative to table sugar = 25% less sweet

Maple syrup
GI 54

3 calories per gram

14 calories per teaspoon table sugar equivalent *

Pure maple syrup has a moderate effect on blood glucose levels. It is a little sweeter than table sugar, but it has fewer calories.

Sweetness relative to table sugar = 10% more sweet

Polydextrose
GI 7

1 calorie per gram

6 calories per teaspoon table sugar equivalent*

Polydextrose has very little effect on blood glucose levels. It is not sweet, but it is used as a bulking agent with non-nutritive sweeteners. It has only one-third the number of calories as table sugar, but it may have a laxative effect if eaten in large quantities.

Sweetness relative to table sugar = not sweet

Table sugar (sucrose)
GI 68

4 calories per gram

16 calories per teaspoon table sugar equivalent*

Also known as superfine sugar, brown sugar, raw sugar, confectioner's sugar

Sucrose or table sugar is the most common sweetener eaten in North America. Despite popular misconceptions, when eaten, it causes blood glucose levels to rise at a moderate rate.

Sweetness = 100%

Xylitol
GI 21

3 calories per gram

14 calories per teaspoon table sugar equivalent*

Xylitol is a sugar alcohol that has essentially no effect on blood glucose levels. It is as sweet as sugar and has fewer calories, but it may have a laxative effect and cause gas and diarrhea if consumed in large quantities.

Sweetness relative to table sugar = 100%

Non-nutritive sweeteners

Acesulphame potassium or Acesulphame K GI 0 0 calories per gram 0 calories per teaspoon table sugar equivalent *	Acesulphame K is hundreds of times sweeter than sugar, has no effect on blood glucose levels, and doesn't provide any calories because it is not absorbed into the body. Sweetness relative to table sugar = 200 times more
Aspartame GI 0 4 calories per gram 0.3 calories per teaspoon table sugar equivalent* Brand names: Nutrasweet, Equal, Equal Spoonful	Aspartame is a couple of hundred times sweeter than sugar and has essentially no effect on blood glucose levels. Because it is a protein, it does provide some calories, but because it is very sweet, you only use it in small amounts. Sweetness relative to table sugar = 150–250 times more *WARNING: Aspartame should not be used by people with phenylketonuria.*
Neotame GI 0 4 calories per gram 0 calories per teaspoon table sugar equivalent*	Neotame is many thousands of times sweeter than sugar and has essentially no effect on blood glucose levels. Because it is a protein, it does provide some calories, but because it is extremely sweet, it is only used in tiny amounts. Sweetness relative to table sugar = 7,000–13,000 times more. While Neotame is approved by the FDA, it is not currently found in any foods or beverages.

Saccharin GI 0 0 calories per gram 0 calories per teaspoon table sugar equivalent* Brand names: Sweet'n'Low, Sugar Twin	Saccharin is hundreds of times sweeter than sugar, has no effect on blood glucose levels and is not metabolised by the human body. Sweetness relative to table sugar = 300–500 times more
Sucralose GI 0 0 calories per gram 0 calories per teaspoon table sugar equivalent* Brand name: Splenda	Sucralose is hundreds of times sweeter than sugar, has no effect on blood glucose levels and does not provide any calories because it is not absorbed into the body. Sweetness relative to table sugar = 400–600 times more

* The number of calories in the volume of alternative sweetener that provides the equivalent sweetness to 1 teaspoon of table sugar

STEP 2:
BE ACTIVE EVERY DAY

Physical activity is one of the cornerstones of managing diabetes and prediabetes.

Chapter 16
Activate your day

It doesn't really matter who you are, or what type of diabetes you have: if you want to be around and in good shape to enjoy your life, your family and your friends, you have to get some exercise.

"I'm active," you say. "I'm on the go all day, walking here and there, in and out of the car, up and down stairs, doing the housework, always busy."

That's great for starters. But what we're talking about here is deliberate muscle movement sessions that add up to at least 150 minutes of physical activity a week, plus making being active and exercising regularly a way of life.

In this chapter we set out the benefits of exercise to get you motivated; and to get you on the move we discuss the kinds of activities you might do and the precautions you need to take when you are doing them, including managing your food and medication during exercise.

If you're already exercising regularly, that's great, but could you do more, or try something different? Whatever the case, you'll find lots of practical ideas here.

There are really only two requirements when it comes to exercise.
One is that you do it.
The other is that you continue to do it.

Why push yourself to exercise?

Exercising muscles need fuel and the fuel they need most is glucose. So as soon as you start moving your muscles they'll start burning up glucose. First they'll use their own stores of glucose (that's glycogen); then they'll call on the liver for some of its stores, all the time drawing the glucose out of the blood and lowering your blood glucose levels.

Here are some of the other benefits (in no particular order) you can get from regular exercise:

- More energy
- Better sleep
- A better mood: exercise produces feel-good chemicals in the brain called endorphins, which will help you cope better with stress
- Better digestion
- Improved immunity
- Stronger bones
- Increased insulin sensitivity: exercise increases the number, sensitivity and binding capacity of insulin receptors
- Lower blood pressure
- Less of the bad cholesterol (LDL) and more of the good (HDL)
- Better circulation so less risk of diabetic complications (including impotence)
- Better weight management and less body fat. After about 30 minutes of continuous exercise the body turns to using fatty acids as a fuel. This clears fats out of your blood and gets some movement happening in the flabby parts
- Fewer hospital admissions or visits to the doctor, and
- Fewer pills to take—medications related to diabetes, blood pressure and cholesterol could be reduced.

Plus, you'll be able to do things you haven't done for years, such as climb a flight of stairs without puffing.

And don't underestimate the positive impact on those around you— you'll be a role model for your family, friends and colleagues!

Activating your day

Start with extra incidental activity

Having to do 30 minutes of exercise every day of the week can seem impossible. What? How? Before thinking about more serious exercise, work on increasing your incidental activity.

Incidental activity means the short bouts of physical activity of 5–10 minutes you accumulate as part of your normal daily routines—making the bed, doing chores, walking to the bus stop, running out for a coffee, parking the car and walking to the store or office. If you make a conscious effort to increase this kind of physical activity in your day, it eventually becomes second nature. Just by adding a little more each day, you will have accumulated the benefits of more exercise by the end of the week.

**Think of incidental activity as an opportunity,
not an inconvenience.**

Here's how, with just a little extra effort, you can build more incidental activity into your life and reap the benefits. You have probably seen lists like this before—we aren't inventing the wheel here. Use our suggestions as a start, then add your own ideas:

- Use the stairs instead of taking the elevator
- Don't stand still on the escalator—walk up or down (holding the rail)

- Take the long way around whenever you can—running down to the corner store, getting a drink from the office water cooler, going to the bathroom
- Make the time to walk the children or grandchildren to school
- Meet your friends for a walk rather than coffee and cake
- Walk the dog instead of throwing tennis balls for it to chase and retrieve
- Get rid of the leaf blower (your neighbors will thank you) and rake the leaves or sweep the yard, and
- Park the car 10 minutes away and walk to the corner store, ATM, post office or dry cleaners: it all adds up.

Getting more serious about exercise

Here are two tips to help you activate your day:

1. Set a schedule, set a reminder, and stick to it! Make the commitment to exercise just the way you make any other important appointment. Remember, habits are developed through practice, and
2. Find a pleasant setting for exercise because this will help keep you motivated. Try a park near work where you can walk, or find a clean, comfortable fitness center, a walking buddy, a smartphone, iPod or radio with earphones, etc.

Before you begin, have a medical checkup.

If you're planning on doing anything more vigorous than brisk walking, you should have a medical checkup first. Now's the time to talk to your doctor about the type of exercise you have in mind and whether or not it is safe for you. Because everyone with prediabetes or diabetes has an increased risk of heart disease, your doctor may want you to do an exercise stress test.

If you have:

Proliferative retinopathy (a non-inflammatory disease of the retina), strenuous exercise or excessive straining is **not recommended** because it increases the risk of hemorrhage (bleeding) in the vitreous space in the eye. If you have had laser photo-coagulation therapy because of your retinopathy, wait 3–6 months before starting or resuming your exercise program.

Peripheral neuropathy (this causes loss of sensation in the feet), avoid weight-bearing exercise because of the danger of injury to your feet. If the condition is mild, suitable footwear can give you enough protection, but alternative exercises such as swimming, cycling, rowing or arm exercises should be considered.

Getting advice on exercise

Exercise specialists such as physiotherapists, exercise physiologists and personal trainers can create an individualized program to suit your needs. Make sure a personal trainer is qualified to work with people who have prediabetes, diabetes or other health problems.

How often should you exercise, and for how long?

For general health, we'd suggest you aim to do 30–60 minutes of exercise most days. If you prefer, you can break this into two or three 15- or 20-minute sessions. For weight loss, research suggests that you need to do 150–300 minutes of moderate intensity exercise each week.

For maximum benefits, leave no more than two days between exercise sessions because the effect of aerobic exercise on insulin sensitivity lasts only 24–72 hours, depending on the duration and intensity of what you do.

To increase your muscle strength and size, do some resistance exercises 2–3 times a week (not on consecutive days); to maintain strength, once a week is enough. Don't worry—you won't end up looking like a bodybuilder unless you spend many hours each day in the gym. But a little bit of extra muscle will help you achieve two important goals for people with prediabetes or diabetes. It will:

- Increase your metabolic rate, and
- Decrease your insulin resistance.

How intense should exercise be?

Lower intensity exercise (exercise that doesn't get you to more than 50 percent of your maximum heartrate) is effective for weight loss. During light exercise, the body uses a larger percentage of fat than glucose (carbohydrate) as a fuel. If you haven't just eaten, the fat is drawn from your body's own stores. As the intensity increases, the body relies more on carbohydrate. A higher intensity (around 75 percent of your maximum heartrate) will be effective for increasing your fitness. For more specific advice on what exercise intensity is best for you, see an exercise specialist.

Measuring the intensity of exercise

There are two ways to do this:

- Monitoring your pulse (heartrate), and
- The simple "talk test."

Monitoring your pulse

Measure your pulse rate with a pulsemeter or by using your wristwatch—this will give you the beats per minute. Then aim for 50–75 percent of your maximum heartrate. Your maximum heartrate is 220 minus your age. For example, if you are 50 years old, here's how you would calculate the number of beats per minute you need to achieve:

1. 50 percent of your maximum heartrate

220 – 50 (age) = 170

170 x 50/100 = 85 beats per minute

2. 75 percent of your maximum heartrate:

220 – 50 (age) = 170

170 x 75/100 = 128 beats per minute

3. When you exercise, aim to keep your heartrate between 85 and 128 beats per minute.

Talk test

The "talk test" means exercising at a pace where you are breathing harder than usual but you can still carry on a conversation comfortably.

When is the best time to exercise?

We're frequently asked this. The unspoken words behind this question are, "When will I burn up the most body fat?"

The best time to exercise is when you can best fit it in. Look for a fairly regular time slot most days. For a lot of people this ends up being first thing in the morning, before the other activities of the day interrupt. But the connection between your head and the pillow can be really strong. Lunchtime exercise sessions can be a great way of destressing from a hectic morning and boosting your energy levels in the afternoon. Even 15–20 minutes here can be a useful regular addition.

In the evening you might have more time available, but there are dangers. Do not sit down in front of the TV or watch a movie until you've done your exercise. If you do, you're gone. Your energy levels are likely to be pretty low at this time, which is great for sleeping but not good for leaping off the couch. If you exercise strenuously, make sure you allow for some wind-down time before bed, or getting to sleep can be difficult.

The length of time you spend on one exercise session will vary depending on your current fitness. If you're just starting out on an exercise program, you might begin with bouts of 10 minutes. The aim should be to get up to 30 minutes a session. If you're exercising comfortably for 30 minutes and want to go even further, you may decide to increase this to 45 or 60 minutes.

If you don't use it, you lose it: a physically inactive adult can expect to lose 3–5 percent of muscle mass and strength per decade after the age of 40.

Types of exercise

What you do is going to depend on how long you've been logged onto the couch. If your body talks back when you try to move it, high-impact activities aren't for you. Swimming, cycling or rowing might be better choices.

For optimal physical fitness, your exercise program ought to include two main types of exercise—aerobic exercise and strength or resistance exercise. Combining the two forms of exercise will have added benefits for diabetes management. Also, stretching, yoga, tai chi and pilates-type exercises will increase your flexibility and balance, and increase your freedom of movement. They are also great for relaxation.

While in general there are three different types of exercise—aerobic, flexibility and resistance/strength—many forms of exercise involve more than one type, and some involve all three. Cycling, for example, is primarily an aerobic exercise, but it also involves resistance training for the legs, as they have to push against a force. Yoga is usually thought of as primarily improving flexibility, yet holding the poses involves a good deal of strength training, using your body weight as resistance.

Aerobic exercise such as walking, running, swimming or cycling gives your heart and lungs a good workout. So it's a great way to get some freshly oxygenated blood pumped through your blood vessels and boost your circulation. Aerobic exercises are also the most efficient way to burn fat. "Aerobic" means "with oxygen," so it is literally any activity that increases your heartrate and breathing.

Strength or resistance exercise

Strength or resistance exercises, such as sit-ups, squats or using weights or resistance bands, will shape and tone your muscles and improve your muscular strength and body composition (decreased fat and more muscle). This kind of exercise is making your muscles work against a resistance or weight. The resistance may be dumb-bells, a resistance elastic band or even your own body weight (as in squats).

Nearly all people who have diabetes can incorporate upper-body strength training with light weights and high repetitions: 1–3 sets working each of the major muscle groups with 8–10 repetitions in each set, for instance.

More strenuous strength training may be acceptable for young people who have diabetes, but it is not recommended for older people or those who have longstanding diabetes.

Strength training is *not* for you if you have:

- Long-term diabetes complications
- Unstable angina (heart pain)
- Uncontrolled hypertension (high blood pressure)
- Uncontrolled dysrhythmia (irregular heartbeat)
- Hypertrophic cardiomyopathy (swollen heart muscles), and/or
- Certain stages of retinopathy.

Benefits of strength training

A recent study (reported in the *Journal of the Amercian Medical Association*) involving nearly 500 men followed for 12 years showed that the reduction in coronary heart disease risk associated with weight training was as good as that from aerobic activities such as running, rowing and walking.

Strength training decreases both total and intra-abdominal (inside the belly) body fat, and—very importantly—helps maintain lean body mass (which would usually be lost when this kind of training is included as part of a weight loss regimen). Very importantly, increased lean body mass is associated with improved insulin sensitivity. Resting metabolic rate is also related to levels of lean body mass. So if you do enough resistance training to increase your muscle mass, you will also get the added bonus of increasing your resting metabolic rate.

As well as the benefits for blood glucose levels, resistance exercise normalizes blood pressure in people with elevated (but not high) blood pressure. Strength training has traditionally not been recommended for people with high blood pressure, but a recent analysis of clinical trials has shown that people with high blood pressure that is treated will also benefit from strength training and that it can be done safely.

Another important finding for people with diabetes and prediabetes is that resistance training improves blood fats. When you look at all the benefits of resistance exercise, it's clear that it is a great all-round activity for people with diabetes.

And that's not all. Strength training also:

- Increases bone mineral density
- Reduces the risk for falls, and
- Reduces pain and improves functioning in osteoarthritis.

The 3 phases of a typical exercise session

1. Warming up (5 minutes): this prepares your body for more strenuous activity and helps prevent injuries. Try gentle walking, cycling, swinging arms, etc.
2. Activity phase: this includes either aerobic and/or resistance exercises. This is the period of more intense aerobic exercise. Try brisk walking, cycling, dancing, stair climbing or even heavy gardening. This will pump up your heartrate and your breathing rate. You might then include some strengthening resistance exercises such as push-ups, lunges or squats—with or without weights—and some for balance, such as side leg raising or standing on one foot for as long as you can.
3. Cooling down (5 minutes): this could include some stretching after your session. Try touching your toes, reaching for the sky, neck stretching. This keeps you flexible and decreases your chances of injury. It also dissipates lactic acid which is formed by exercising muscles and gradually returns your body to its normal state. This prevents pooling of blood in the arms and legs, which could cause fainting.

Building up the aerobic activity phase from 15 minutes to 30–40 minutes will maximize the health benefits.

Walking

One of the most popular forms of physical activity is simply going for a walk—whether it's around your house or garden, the neighborhood, the park, or perhaps along the beach or a trail. Walking is a surprisingly effective form of exercise for people with diabetes or those trying to prevent it.

A recent study reported in the American Diabetes Association's prestigious journal *Diabetes Care* provides convincing proof that regular walking can provide significant health benefits for very little cost. A group of nearly 200 people with type 2 diabetes were given physical activity counseling every three months for two years. Some took it more seriously than others. The researchers found that those walking 1–3 miles (2,400–6,400 steps) *more* than usual each day achieved the most benefits for their diabetes.

Moving more and sitting less

In recent years researchers have linked sitting for long periods of time with serious health risk. In fact a 2012 analysis of studies found that people who sat for the longest periods of time each day were twice as likely to have diabetes or heart disease, as those who sat the least.

Prolonged sitting impairs the normal function of arteries in distributing blood flow. This has detrimental effects on common parameters like blood pressure but may also turn down the genes and enzymes involved in fat and glucose metabolism.

Sitting for too long is not the same as exercising too little. Working out in the gym for 30 minutes a day doesn't undo the effect of sitting for the rest of the day, but intermittent movement can.

By interspersing periods of sitting with brief periods of activity such as 5–10 minutes of walking or stair-climbing once every hour can prevent the decline in arterial function.

Exercise, eating and
your blood glucose levels

If you don't take insulin or blood glucose-lowering medication and your blood glucose level is normally well controlled, you shouldn't need to do extra checks or eat differently when you exercise.

If your blood glucose level is less than 5.5 mmol/l (99 mg/dL) and you take insulin, aim to eat 15–20g of carbohydrate 15–30 minutes before you exercise. (The same applies to children with a level less than 7 mmol/l, or 126 mg/dL). Recheck your blood glucose levels again 30 minutes into the exercise to prevent hypoglycemia. Finally, check your blood glucose levels immediately after you have finished exercising (see Chapter 17).

Generally, exercise will lower blood glucose levels, but it can have the opposite effect sometimes. Exercising muscles are hungry for glucose and will use up their own stores, then search the bloodstream for more. When blood glucose levels start to drop, the liver releases its stores, and if they run out, it can convert protein to glucose. This glucose can be quickly released into the blood. Sometimes, if you do really strenuous exercise, or you are a little unwell, your blood glucose levels can go high when you exercise, due to the release of stress hormones such as adrenaline. If you have enough insulin, they will drop again over time, as the muscles and liver replenish their glucose stores.

Chapter 17
Exercise: Keeping it going

Exercise: getting started and keeping it going

Depending on how much of a couch potato you've been, it's going to take time to get fit. Initially there'll be some discomfort or breathlessness, and you'll just want to stop. In time, breathing will become easier, and you'll develop a feeling of physical wellbeing. Finally you'll attain psychological fitness—exhilaration, mental relaxation and real enjoyment of the physical effort. Here are some tips for when the going gets tough:

- Try something different. Don't do the same exercise every session: ride a bicycle one day, walk the next, and swim another day. This gives you variety in your routine and reduces the risk of injury by avoiding straining the same muscles all the time.
- Record what you do and monitor your progress: show your notes to the members of your diabetes management team so they know how hard you have been working.
- Set goals: setting specific goals for yourself and then evaluating how you are doing is a great way to keep on track. Remember to write

them down so that they are more tangible. But be realistic; unrealistic goals can work against you.

- If time is tight, make your exercise time productive: you could prop up your newspaper or iPad on your stationary bike, or park your treadmill in front of the TV so you can watch the news or make phone calls while you cycle/walk/jog.

- Get an exercise buddy: if someone is there waiting for you, you are far more likely to keep on track. If you can afford it, you could get a personal trainer.

- Reward yourself: a good way to keep your motivation high is to reward yourself when you accomplish a goal. Give yourself a new item of training gear, a book, a visit to the movies, a massage—anything healthy that will keep you motivated.

Exercise tips

- If you don't need to lose weight, increase your food intake to match your increased exercise. This is particularly important during strenuous activity, when you need to replace the energy you have burned. Always have some fast-acting carbohydrate on hand too.

- Drink water before, during and after exercise. Water is the best form of fluid replacement. Unless you are performing extreme endurance sports, sports drinks are not necessary. A good habit to establish is to have a large glass (10–16 oz) of water 15 minutes before exercise. Have another 8 oz glass of water for every 15 minutes of exercise, and have another large glass when you have finished.

- Exercise regularly, ideally at the same time each day.

- Be consistent with exercise and meal times and insulin injections.

- Plan on adjusting your dose of insulin according to what you are going to do. This is particularly relevant if you are over-weight. Take care not to exaggerate the calories burned during exercise: to burn up just 1 slice of bread (75 calories, on average), you need to walk for about 20 minutes or jog for 10 minutes.
- Avoid heavy exercise when your insulin action is at its peak.
- Use your stomach rather than your limbs for injecting. Insulin injected into muscle will be absorbed very quickly and could lower your blood glucose too much. You may need an extra 15–20g of carbohydrate during bouts of vigorous exercise that last an hour or more.
- If you are planning on doing a particular activity regularly (and we hope you are), it's a good idea to experiment with the activity around the same time of day on at least three occasions to see how your blood glucose levels respond. Test before, immediately after and then again 6–8 hours after exercising.

Exercising safely

It is a good idea to do the following:
- Carry some quickly absorbed carbohydrate, such as a sweetened drink or gummy bears, and try to exercise with someone who knows you have diabetes, not alone
- Have a contact—someone who knows where you are, or who exercises with you—or keep a phone with you
- Wear an ID bracelet or necklace so that if something does happen while you are alone, first responders will be able to help more quickly

- Replace fluids
- If you need to take insulin, look out for low blood sugar symptoms during and up to 24 hours afterward, and
- Protect your feet by wearing good-fitting shoes and cotton socks.

You Should Stop:
- At the first sign of injury
- If you feel light-headed
- At the first hint of low blood sugar
- If you experience severe shortness of breath
- If you have any pain or pressure in your chest, or
- If you experience any loss of balance or dizziness.

Reducing the risk of hypoglycemia

If you take insulin and/or sulfonylurea medications such as Chlorpropamide (Diabinese), Glipizide (GlipiZIDE XL, Glucotrol, Glucotrol XL), Glyburide (Glynase and DiaBeta) or Glimepiride (Amaryl), you are more likely to develop hypoglycemia or "have a hypo" when you are physically active—particularly for prolonged periods.

It can also be more difficult to recognize the symptoms of hypo-glycemia when you are physically active because the usual warning signs—sweating, rapid heartbeat and shaking—can be easily confused with normal responses to exercise. This is why it is so important to monitor your blood glucose before, during and after activity.

If you do have low blood sugar when exercising, one carbohydrate exchange (approximately 15g) will raise your blood glucose levels rapidly.

What kind of carbohydrate is best when you are exercising?

For practical purposes, when you are doing less than 1½ hours of exercise at one time, the type of carbohydrate you eat does not really need to be different from what you eat on days when you are not exercising. It is only when you are exercising for more than 90 minutes at a time that it seems to make a significant difference.

Exercise, blood glucose and carbohydrate quantity

Activity and duration	Blood sugar mg/dL	Carbohydrate quantity
Light (walking for 30 minutes)	less than 108 more than 108	1–2 exchanges* generally nothing
Moderate (swimming, cycling, running, brisk walking, surfing for 1 hour)	108–180 180–270 more than 270	1–2 exchanges generally nothing if unwell, do not exercise and check ketones
Strenuous (hockey, football, cycling, continuous swimming, running, endurance sports, hiking for 1 hour or more)	less than 108 108–180 180–270 more than 270	3 exchanges 2–3 exchanges 0–1 exchange if unwell, do not exercise and check ketones

Adapted from *Caring for Diabetes in Children and Adolescents: A Parent's Manual*

* See page 59

GI and exercise

As we explained in Chapter 10, low GI foods deliver a slower, more sustained release of glucose into the bloodstream, and high GI foods cause a fast and high glucose response, which means that they will be more immediately available.

Research has shown that using low GI foods before an activity can improve performance. Specifically, you can perform an activity more quickly or keep on doing the activity for 20 percent longer, compared to high GI foods or meals.

Carbohydrate choices for sustained physical activity

Before and after activity	Low GI foods
Before: to produce sustained blood glucose	pasta, yogurt, milk, apples, dried apricots
After: to improve muscle glycogen repletion	heavy grain breads, rolled oats, All-Bran, baked beans, 100% fruit juice
During activity	**High GI foods**
To maintain glucose for working muscles	sports drinks such as Gatorade

STEP 3:
MANAGE YOUR WEIGHT

Excess body weight is going to make your blood glucose levels more difficult to control. Extra body fat, particularly around the waist, contributes to insulin resistance—the condition where your cells are "deaf" to the effect of insulin. Also, excess weight makes exercising difficult, increases your blood pressure and increases your chances of developing diabetic complications. So managing body weight is an issue for lots of people with diabetes.

Chapter 18
How to achieve
your weight loss goals

Weight "control" comes easily for some. Without any real conscious effort, they maintain a fairly stable weight throughout their adult life, thanks mainly to good in-built regulatory control.

Weight management shouldn't be an issue for the human body. We are designed with a whole host of systems that regulate energy intake and expenditure in order to maintain a steady state. But something has gone wrong, and for many people, excess weight gain occurs.

So what do you do about it? Well, losing a little weight, or at least stabilizing it, is a priority. But as we said in Chapter 6, you don't have to be "the biggest loser." Setting attainable weight loss goals is the key.

We are not talking about going on a traditional restrictive diet. The best way to achieve your weight loss goals (and maintain your new weight) is through gradual change, including changing the way you eat, and increasing your physical activity. In **Part 3: Living with diabetes and prediabetes and the metabolic syndrome**, we have put together a series of eating plans for people with diabetes and prediabetes.

Along with making sure you move more, we focus on the following types of changes:

- Reducing how much you eat (but we promise you won't feel hungry)

- Cutting back on saturated fats and cholesterol
- Modifying your carbohydrate intake
- Eating more regularly
- Moderating your protein intake
- Eating more (yes, more) healthy foods like fruit and vegetables of all sorts except most potatoes, and
- Cutting back on salt.

Why restrictive diets don't work

If you are overweight, chances are you have tried a number of diets over the years. At best, a restrictive diet will reduce your calorie intake (while you stick to it!); at worst it will change your body composition for the fatter. Why? When you lose weight through severely restricting your food intake, you lose some of your body's muscle mass. Over the years, this type of dieting will change your body composition to less muscle and proportionately more fat, making weight control increasingly difficult. Your body's engine will require less and less energy to keep it running. In fact, the majority of people who lose weight by "strict" dieting will regain it.

Restricting food also has adverse psychological consequences. Self-imposed dieting and starvation tend to result in:

- Eating binges when food is around
- A preoccupation with food and eating, and
- A heightened emotional response to food.

**Remember, most people don't fail to lose weight;
they fail to maintain weight loss.**

What we know about weight management

There is no single approach to weight management that guarantees success (despite what the advertisements for the latest "miracle" weight-loss program claim). There is no magic bullet. Being overweight or obese is a complex condition with many causes—and sadly, a very low "cure" rate.

While research regularly gives us new insight into the complexities of "obesity genes," "appetite hormones," and neurotransmitters that affect eating behavior, what we know about weight management can actually be stated quite simply.

First of all, weight loss diets alone stand little chance of success. So what does help?

- Consuming foods that provide fewer calories per bite, which means more fruit and vegetables
- Exercise, especially for maintaining weight loss
- Modifying your behavior so that you become more aware of what you eat, why and when, and
- An intensive lifestyle change program that includes regular physical activity, reduced calorie intake, support and frequent contact with a health professional (such as a dietitian). As few as six biweekly visits, either face-to-face or in a group, may make all the difference; it is good to know you are not alone.

How often you eat (one or two large meals or six small ones of equal energy density) makes little difference to the rate of weight loss.

We also know that not all foods are created equal. Research has shown that the type of food you give your body determines what it is going to burn and what it is going to store as body fat and that certain foods are more satisfying to the appetite than others. Low GI foods (fruit and vegetables, low GI cereal grains and products made from them, legumes, nuts and lower fat dairy foods) give you the edge. They fill you up and keep you satisfied for longer, and they help you burn more body fat and less muscle.

Exercise for weight loss and weight maintenance

How much exercise do you need to do to get weight off and keep it off?

Although it varies, the short answer is, more than you think. The best evidence comes from the US National Weight Control Registry. This includes the data of approximately 5,000 people who have lost an average of 65 lbs and maintained their weight loss for at least 1 year (the average of those on the register is 5 years). These people report doing the equivalent of approximately 7 hours per week of moderate intensity exercise. This means something close to really brisk walking for at least one hour a day, **every day**.

Energy in—what you actually eat

However, if you are obese, exercise alone is unlikely to be enough to bring about much weight loss (partly because extra physical activity is so difficult and is very easily counterbalanced). Most obese people have to reduce their energy intake as well.

There is not one ideal "diet" that will be right for everyone. Most weight loss diets are based on a particular nutrient composition, and the potential combinations are endless. Low-fat and low carbohydrate (including low sugar) diets have been popular choices in recent years and high protein diets are still popular.

If you accept that you have to create an energy deficit, the solution is really to find the easiest way to do this, a strategy that you can live with. And there are lots of strategies:

- **Strategy 1**: most people don't find it easy simply to eat less of their favorite foods. But some types of foods can make it easier to eat less. Foods that are high in protein or low GI carbohydrate are more satisfying and make you feel fuller for longer than fat- and carbohydrate-rich foods with a high GI.
- **Strategy 2**: don't eat less in terms of volume, but eat foods with a lower energy density (fewer calories per bite). Fruits and vegetables, for example, have very few calories, but because they are bulky and fibrous, they can be very filling. The same could be said about low GI wholegrain and high fiber cereals, which are more filling and less energy dense than their refined counterparts.
- **Strategy 3**: focus on eating a lower fat diet to reduce your calorie intake without necessarily eating less. Because fat provides more calories per gram than any other nutrient, reducing fats will help lower your calorie intake.

The importance of a good night's sleep

US researchers analyzing data of 18,000 adults in the National Health and Nutrition Examination Survey found a correlation between BMI (body mass index) and hours of sleep per night. Those who got less than 4 hours of sleep a night were 73 percent more likely to be obese than those who slept 7–9 hours a night. In a separate study of 924 adults, researchers determined that 2 hours less sleep per week amounted to an increase in BMI of 10.

They're still at a loss to explain how sleep helps our weight, but there are lots of theories. It may be related to lower production of the hormone leptin (a natural appetite suppressant) with sleep deprivation. In the meantime, it's a good reason to make sure you get enough shut-eye.

If you need to lose weight, how much should you aim to lose?

Setting attainable goals is extremely important. You can achieve significant health benefits by losing just 5 percent of your body weight if you were overweight or obese when you were first diagnosed with diabetes.

For some people, losing this amount (and maintaining the loss) is easy, though it needs some fairly major changes in eating habits. For others, losing even 10 lbs and maintaining that loss is very difficult. If this is the case for you, it might be more realistic to simply aim for no weight gain (because we all tend to get fatter as we get older).

Weight management has two different phases—losing weight and maintaining the weight loss. During the weight loss phase, a reasonable aim (unless you are very overweight) might be to lose 3–5 lbs a month over a period of about 3 months. After losing 10–15 lbs your weight will probably plateau.

Maintaining your weight loss, give or take a pound or two, over the next 3-month period is crucial in terms of helping you consolidate your diet and exercise habits. Giving your body time to adjust to a lower weight takes the pressure off and increases your chances of maintaining your new weight.

If you succeed in losing 5–10 percent of your body weight but want to lose more, only try to do it after a period of weight maintenance. Using an alternating "weight loss/weight maintenance" strategy increases your chances of success in the long run.

What's a good rate of weight loss?

3–5 lbs a month

What does it take to lose about 1 pound a week?

In theory, to achieve weight loss of about 1 pound a week you need to reduce your daily energy intake by about 680 calories a day—assuming you haven't increased your physical activity expenditure.

What's your BMI?

Your body mass index (BMI) is a measure of your weight in relation to your height. In Caucasian people, a BMI greater than 25 is classified as overweight, and above 30 as obese. Different cut-offs apply for people from other ethnic backgrounds, and more muscular people should use a cut-off of 27 for being overweight. People of Asian origin should use a cut-off of 23.

To calculate your BMI, here is the formula:

$$\text{weight (lb)} / [\text{height (in)}]^2 \times 703$$

Calculate BMI by dividing weight in pounds (lbs) by height in inches (in) squared and multiplying by a conversion factor of 703.

Example: Weight = 150 lbs, Height = 5'5" (65")
Calculation: $[150 \div (65)^2] \times 703 = 24.96$
Source: cdc.gov

But you don't have to do the math. There are some handy online BMI calculators. Try **www.nhlbi.nih.gov/health/educational/lose_wt/ BMI/bmicalc.htm**

BMI cut-offs for Asian people

	Overweight	Obesity
China	24	29
China (Hong Kong)	23	27
Indonesia	24	26
Japan	25	30
Singapore	22	27
Thailand (urban)	25	30
Thailand (rural)	27	31

STEP 4:
DON'T SMOKE.
IF YOU DO, QUIT

Smoking increases the risk of developing type 2 diabetes—the more you smoke, the greater your risk. There are lots of options to help you kick the habit, from nicotine patches and gums, to medication, counseling, even hypnosis.

Be aware that nicotine patches may raise blood glucose levels in some people with diabetes. Talk to your doctor, diabetes educator or other members of your healthcare team for advice.

Chapter 19
Smoking and diabetes complications

Smoking damages and constricts our blood vessels, decreasing the flow of blood throughout our body so that less oxygen is delivered to our vital organs and tissues. Smoking also raises blood glucose levels, making diabetes harder to manage. Finally, smoking increases our cholesterol and triglyceride levels.

So a smoker's risk of developing heart and blood vessel diseases such as stroke and peripheral vascular disease are substantially increased. For example, it has been estimated that people with diabetes who smoke have at least three times the risk of developing heart disease of a person with diabetes who's a nonsmoker, and they are much more likely to die if they do suffer a heart attack.

The damage caused by smoking to the blood vessels and circulation also leads to poor wound healing, which can lead to leg and foot infections, and then lead to amputation—95 percent of the people with diabetes who need amputations are smokers.

If you smoke and you have diabetes, you are also more likely to get nerve damage and kidney disease, and you'll get colds and respiratory infections more easily, and these cause fluctuations in blood glucose levels.

If all these problems are not a big enough incentive to stop, smoking can also increase the risk of impotence, which is a significant problem for men with diabetes even if they don't smoke!

Smoking just one cigarette reduces the body's ability to use insulin by 15 percent! Once you stop smoking, the insulin resistance does not start to improve until 10–12 hours later.

Smoking and food

Smoking also influences dietary habits.

- Smokers tend to eat less fruit and vegetables than nonsmokers (and so they get less of the protective antioxidant plant compounds that these foods provide), and
- Smokers tend to eat more fat and more salt than nonsmokers.

These characteristics of the smoker's diet may be caused by a desire to seek strong food flavors, which could itself be because smoking blunts your ability to taste. There is only one piece of advice for anyone who smokes: quit.

The benefits of quitting

When you quit smoking, your insulin resistance decreases, and you will have less chance of developing diabetes (if you have prediabetes), and of developing its common complications (such as kidney and nerve damage).

You may also find that you have lower blood glucose and HbA1c levels, lower total and LDL (bad) cholesterol and triglyceride levels, and higher

HDL (good) cholesterol levels. The combined effect will be a lower risk of having a heart attack or stroke.

Once you stop smoking, your insulin requirements may drop by up to 30 percent. So if you are taking diabetes medications or insulin it's very important to monitor your blood glucose levels more frequently when you first quit.

Because of the decrease in insulin resistance, many people with diabetes find their blood glucose levels are significantly lower after they quit. This may mean insulin or medication adjustments—see your doctor, diabetes educator or dietitian for further advice.

Electronic cigarettes

An electronic cigarette or e-cigarette is an electronic inhaler that is used as a substitute for regular smoking. A heating element is used to vaporize a liquid solution—usually containing nicotine. They are usually designed to mimic traditional smoking implements, such as cigarettes or cigars, in their use and appearance. In theory, e-cigarettes should have fewer toxic effects than traditional cigarettes/cigars; however, convincing evidence is lacking, although there is some anecdotal evidence that they are safer than regular cigarettes/cigars, and possibly as safe as other nicotine replacement products.

STEP 5:
LIMIT YOUR CONSUMPTION OF ALCOHOL

One of the things many people ask when first diagnosed with diabetes is, "Can I still have a drink?" In the past, the usual answer was no because it was thought that the sugars in many alcoholic drinks could affect blood glucose levels, and alcohol contributes to weight gain. Alcohol is very high in calories, providing 7 calories per gram (an average drink has 10g of alcohol or more). In fact it is the second most concentrated source of energy in the diet after fat, which provides 9 calories per gram.

We now know that there may be some benefits to enjoying an occasional glass of wine or beer if you have diabetes or prediabetes.

**Whatever your reason for having a drink,
the key message for everybody, whether you have diabetes,
prediabetes or neither, is do it in moderation!**

Chapter 20
Can I still have a drink?

If you are trying to lose weight, it is best to think of alcohol as an indulgence, as "keep for a treat" fare. It may be enjoyable, but it doesn't provide any essential nutrients and it is high in calories.

If you have diabetes or prediabetes, it's important to limit your daily consumption of alcohol. This is because alcohol contributes to weight gain, high triglycerides and high blood pressure, and therefore increases the risk of developing diabetes complications.

If you use insulin or are taking certain blood glucose-lowering medications, such as sulphonylureas or meglitinides, alcohol increases your risk of having low blood sugar for up to 24 hours after you have stopped drinking. This is because alcohol reduces glucose production by the liver and reduces the body's ability to release glucose into the blood. This may also make it harder to treat than usual. Even a small amount of alcohol impairs your ability to detect low blood sugar, and if the people you're drinking with are also drinking, they may not be any help— so beware.

Alcohol and the body

Alcohol affects your body in many different ways. In fact, **excessive consumption is linked to over 60 different medical conditions—so far**. Most of us know that excessive consumption can damage our brain and liver. What many don't know is that it can also damage your stomach and pancreas, and it increases the risk of developing heart disease, stroke, and breast, mouth and throat cancer. For men it has a particularly unfortunate effect on the sex organs, leading to the inability to get and/or sustain an erection despite its ability to increase sexual desire.

Alcohol is "fattening"—the body has no place to store alcohol, so it takes top priority as a source of fuel, sending other fuel sources (food) to storage. This means that if you drink a can of beer with a bag of chips, or have a glass of wine with cheese, your body will "burn" the alcohol first and most likely store the fat from the chips or cheese.

As we said, alcohol is just extra indulgence calories, and, unfortunately, the "beer belly" is now seen in women as well as men. In fact the latest research shows that more women (57 percent) than men (55 percent) have a high waist circumference—a classic sign of eating and drinking to excess.

How much is safe to drink?

Enjoying a moderate amount of alcohol with food will have little effect on your blood glucose levels. Indeed recent research from the University of Sydney suggests that a glass or two of wine with or before a meal may reduce the rise in glucose levels by 25 percent. Contrary to common belief, alcoholic drinks (apart from mixes) don't contain a lot of sugar. A standard drink of regular beer contains only about 7.5g (a rounded teaspoon) of carbohydrate, light beer about 9g and low carb beer an average of 3.5g. Wine and spirits are even lower with standard drinks containing less than 1g of carbohydrate. So it's not the sugar content of alcohol that's the problem, it's the alcohol itself. This is because there's very little carbohydrate in most alcoholic drinks: on average, a 12 fl oz glass of regular beer contains only 12g of carbs per serving; light beer has 6g; a 5 fl oz glass of wine has 4g; and a standard shot of spirits has no carbs.

Moderate drinking is the amount that has been linked with the least risk and greatest benefits. The good news is that research indicates that in general, the level of alcohol consumption associated with the least risk for people with diabetes is the same as that for the rest of the adult population. That is, women should have no more than one standard drink per day and men no more than two standard drinks on any day. It is also a good idea to have at least two alcohol-free days each week.

However, if you are overweight, have poorly managed blood glucose levels, high blood pressure, high triglycerides or other diabetic complications, your diabetes healthcare team may advise you to drink less or not to drink at all.

What is a standard drink?

A standard drink is less than you think! Technically it's an amount that contains roughly 14g of pure alcohol and is equal to:

- 12 fl oz of regular beer, about 5 percent alcohol
- 8 fl oz of malt liquor, about 7 percent alcohol
- 5 fl oz glass of wine, about 12 percent alcohol
- 1.5 fl oz (one shot) of 80 proof spirits, about 40 percent alcohol

It's easy to underestimate the amount you drink, so if you want to stick to the guidelines, learn how much is in a standard drink of whatever types of alcoholic drink you like before you start drinking. Simple ways of doing this include:

- Checking the number of standard drinks listed on the label of the bottle, and

- Measuring out a standard drink with a measuring cup so you know exactly what it looks like.

When you do this, you will probably be surprised by how much your favorite glass actually holds. For example, many wine glasses, when full, may hold almost two standard drinks!

What about mixers?

As we said, alcoholic drinks contain very little carbohydrate, so they have very little impact on blood glucose levels if they are drunk in moderation. However, many people like to mix alcohol with soft drinks, mixers or fruit juices, and standard varieties of all those are high in added sugar. Though moderate amounts of added sugars will not necessarily cause blood glucose levels to rise rapidly, they do contribute to the overall glycemic load of your diet without giving you any vitamins, minerals or fiber. Therefore for many, it may be wiser to simply choose "diet" mixers instead of the "standard" varieties. The following list will help you understand why:

Mixer	Carbohydrate in a 10 fl oz glass
Regular flavored soft drinks	32g
Tonic water	27g
Fruit juice	26g
Cola	22g
Mixer (made with water)	19g
Tomato juice	14g
Diet mixer	3g
Diet soft drinks	0g
Diet tonic water	0g
Soda water	0g
Water	0g

Although low-carb or low-sugar beers have about half the sugar content of regular beer, the difference is only a few grams, which won't make much difference in terms of your blood glucose levels. They are slightly lower in calories but are generally full alcohol so still carry the risk of low blood sugar.

What about premixed drinks?

Many people now have premixed drinks (sometimes called "alcopops" or "coolers") instead of the more traditional beer and wine. Unlike beer and wine, most premixed drinks *do* contain significant amounts of carbohydrate.

Most of the mixers that are used have an intermediate GI (56–69), and in moderation, they are unlikely to cause hyperglycemia (high glucose readings). However, they do give you extra carbohydrate: most contain at least as much as you would find in a slice or two of bread, and some, such as the vodka with lemon, lime and soda, contain a lot more. Take this into account when you plan your meals (and insulin doses, if you take insulin).

Brand	Volume (fl oz)	Energy (cal)	Alcohol (g)	Carbohydrate (g)
Wildberry Schnapps	1	103	6.5	11
Kahlua Mudslide	4	280	12	33.5
Bacardi Classic Cocktails Mojito	4	160	13.7	16
Bud Lite Lime-a-Rita	8	220	14.9	29.1
Jose Cuervo Authentic Classic Lime Margarita	4	139	8	19.4

How does alcohol interact with insulin or blood glucose-lowering medications?

Take extra care when drinking alcohol if you take these medications:

- Sulfonylureas (such as Amaryl, Diabinese, Glucotrol, Micronase, Glynase, Daonil or Rastinon)
- Meglitinides (such as Prandin and Siarlix), or
- Insulin.

The alcohol and the medication can interact and cause hypoglycemia. Sometimes sulfonylureas can interact with alcohol to cause nausea, vomiting or flushing. Speak to your doctor or pharmacist if you are not sure what type of medication you are taking.

Many other medications react with alcohol. If you are taking any, check with your doctor or pharmacist before drinking alcohol.

What should I eat when I'm drinking?

It's a good idea to combine drinking alcohol with food. This will slow the rate of absorption of the alcohol, and thus reduce the degree of intoxication. Lower fat, low GI carbohydrate foods are the least likely to make you store fat—they will release glucose slowly into the bloodstream, reducing the risk of both high and low blood glucose levels.

If you have been drinking during the afternoon or evening, we recommend a low GI snack before going to bed to help maintain your blood glucose levels through the night. A piece of wholegrain toast, a glass of milk, a carton of yogurt or pieces of fruit are good. This is particularly important if you take insulin.

If you take insulin, sulphonylureas or meglitinides, make sure you eat some carbohydrate foods (see ideas below) while you are drinking, to prevent low blood sugar. If you are at a party and food is not available, try using juice, milk or regular soft drink as sources of carbohydrate.

Avoiding low blood sugar is more important in the short term than watching your carbohydrate intake!

Savory snacks	Fruits
Bread	Fruit platter
Microwaved popcorn	Fresh fruit salad
Ryvita	Dried fruit (dates, apricots,
Wholegrain crackers and crispbread	figs, etc.)

Who shouldn't drink alcohol?

If you have a fatty liver, high triglycerides, pancreatitis, advanced neuropathy or any form of liver disease you should not drink any alcohol.

Also, if you are pregnant, planning to have a baby or breastfeeding, we recommend you do not drink any alcohol.

Tips for drinking less

If you think you are drinking too much, try some of the following ideas to help reduce your alcohol intake:

- Drink some water or a diet soft drink before you drink any alcohol, so you are not thirsty when you start.
- Order a glass of wine and a glass of water at the same time.
- Sip your alcoholic drink slowly.
- Drink a non-alcoholic drink after every alcoholic drink (for example water or a diet soft drink).
- Dilute alcohol (make a shandy by diluting your beer with low calorie lemonade, or dilute your wine with soda water for instance).
- Drink low alcohol beer.

Oh no, I think I drank too much . . .

Unfortunately, many people experience a hangover at least once in their lives. The aching head, parched mouth, burning stomach and general feeling of having been hit by a truck often lead to promises of "giving up the booze" . . . well, at least for a few days.

While there is no such thing as a cure for a hangover, there are a number of simple, inexpensive things that you can try to help you get through the day. The main symptoms of a hangover are thought to be due to lack of deep sleep, dehydration, irritation of the digestive tract, loss of B group vitamins in the urine, and decreased blood glucose due to decreased glucose production by the liver. If you think about these individually, you can put together a "recipe" that should at least give you some temporary relief:

Step 1: Replace the fluid you lost. Electrolyte drinks such as Gatorade come in handy here—they help you absorb the fluid more quickly and give you some carbohydrate.

Step 2: Take 2 Tylenol (not aspirin—it may irritate your stomach more) along with the fluids.

Step 3: Have a multi B group vitamin.

Step 4: If you find your blood glucose levels are dropping low, have some low GI carbohydrate (reduced fat milk or yogurt, or fresh fruit, for example). These foods will also give you some extra fluids and help soothe your sore stomach.

Step 5: Avoid caffeinated beverages (coffee, tea, soft drinks and chocolate) because they make you go to the toilet more.

Step 6: Monitor your blood glucose more than usual to ensure you avoid hypoglycemia.

Mocktail, anyone?

Whatever your reason for not drinking alcohol, or reducing your alcohol intake, there are many low alcohol or non-alcoholic alternatives that can help you enjoy the spirit of a social occasion without the side effects.

Very low alcohol beers and wines are available in most supermarkets. Low alcohol beers contain roughly the same amount of carbohydrate as the alcoholic varieties and will have little effect on your blood glucose levels if you drink them in moderation.

Most non-alcoholic wines, on the other hand, are based on grape juice, and give you about 15g of carbohydrate per 3.5 ounce serving. Like most juices, they probably won't cause your blood glucose levels to rise rapidly, but just because they are alcohol free, don't think you can drink them freely!

If you're after a fancy drink without alcoholic side effects try a "mocktail"—an artistically presented blend of non-alcoholic beverages. There are lots of recipes for mocktails on the Internet. Here are some to try:

Mickey Mouse
Glass: highball glass
Mixers: 3 oz orange juice
1 oz diet raspberry syrup
3 oz diet soda
Method: Build over ice
Garnish: 2 cherries on side of glass
Cal = 43; carbohydrates = 9g; alcohol = 0g

Lethal Weapon

Glass: highball glass

Mixers: 7 oz vegetable juice

1 teaspoon chili or Tabasco sauce

Salt and pepper

½ oz lemon juice

Method: Build over ice and stir

Garnish: Celery stalk

Cal = 60; carbohydrates = 10g; alcohol = 0g

Shirley Temple

Glass: highball glass

Mixers: ½ oz grenadine

Diet ginger ale, lemon-lime soda or lemonade

Method: Build over ice

Garnish: Slice of orange with straw

Cal = 38; carbohydrates = 9g; alcohol = 0g

PART 3:

Living with diabetes, prediabetes and the metabolic syndrome

Serving sizes of carbohydrates, proteins and fats

In the next section, we will be providing daily meal guides, based on servings of carbohydrate, proteins and fats. Each of these is based on typical household servings of foods.

How much is a serving?

Within each of the different food groups you will find serving sizes of foods that are nutritionally similar. For example, 1 slice of bread has a similar amount of carbohydrate to ⅓ cup of cooked rice (roughly). Within one group, foods can be swapped or exchanged for another. For example, two servings of *breads, cereals and other starchy foods* could be taken as ⅔ cup of muesli or 1 cup of corn kernels.

C A R B O H Y D R A T E S

Breads, cereals and other starchy foods
1 slice of bread (30–35g)
⅓ cup natural muesli (30–35g)
¼ cup raw rolled oats (30g)
½ cup All-Bran (30–35g)
⅓ cup cooked rice (65g)
⅓ cup pearl barley (65g)
½ large ear of corn (80g)
½ cup (90g) corn kernels
½ cup (75g) cooked pasta or noodles
½ cup (85g) cooked chickpeas, kidney beans, borlotti beans etc.
¾ cup (145g) cooked lentils
1 cup (180g) cooked split peas
¾ cup (110g) diced sweet potato
2 small new potatoes or 1 medium sized (125g)
½ cup (125g) mashed potato

C A R B O H Y D R A T E S

Fruit

1 medium sized piece of fruit (e.g., apple, orange, banana)

2 small pieces of fruit (e.g., apricots, plums, kiwi)

½ cup (120–130g) diced pieces or canned fruit

20g dried fruit (e.g., 1½ tbsp raisins, 6 dates, 6 apricot halves)

4 prunes (30g)

½ cup (150ml) fruit juice

Milk and milk products

1 cup (125ml) low or reduced fat milk

1 cup calcium-fortified soy milk

6.5 oz carton low-fat yogurt

1 cup (250ml) buttermilk

P R O T E I N S

Meat and alternatives

100g raw lean meat or chicken

150g raw fish

100g drained, canned fish

200g tofu or cooked soybeans

2 omega-3 enriched eggs

60g reduced fat hard cheese

4 slices (pre-packed) (84g) reduced fat processed cheese

F A T S

Fat-rich foods

2 tsp mono- or polyunsaturated margarine

2 tsp mono- or polyunsaturated oil

3 tsp peanut butter

20g nuts

1–2 tbsp oil-based salad dressing

¼ (50g) avocado

Vegetables

½ cup of cooked vegetables

1 cup of raw leafy salad vegetables

1 cup vegetable soup or pure vegetable juice

MANAGING PREDIABETES AND THE METABOLIC SYNDROME

"Just a touch of sugar" is how prediabetes is often described, which is why, not surprisingly, so many people think it's not such a big deal. But it is potentially a very big deal. If you have prediabetes, you're also more likely to have more of the risk factors for heart disease and stroke, including high blood pressure and high levels of LDL (bad) cholesterol, thanks to insulin resistance. And you are more likely to develop full-blown type 2 diabetes within 5–10 years.

As we explained in Chapter 3, if you have prediabetes, it means your body doesn't handle blood glucose as well as it used to or should, but your blood glucose levels are not high enough yet to say that you have type 2 diabetes. It's a step toward type 2 diabetes and heart disease, but it's not necessarily a one-way ticket.

Chapter 21
Living with prediabetes

What can you do about prediabetes?

Plenty.

Lifestyle changes—moderate weight loss, healthy eating and regular physical activity—will go a long way. In fact three out of five people (as shown in the US Diabetes Prevention Program) with prediabetes can prevent it developing into type 2 diabetes simply by adopting these lifestyle changes.

Taking steps to avoid diabetes

- Aim for moderate weight loss by reducing your calorie intake
- Lower your saturated fat intake
- Boost your omega-3 intake
- Lower the GI of your diet
- Increase your fiber intake, and
- Get regular physical activity.

Aim for moderate weight loss

For most people with prediabetes, the first priority has to be reducing body weight. You don't have to lose a lot of weight for it to help. Research has shown that people with prediabetes who lose 5–10 percent of their body weight at diagnosis can prevent or delay the onset of type 2 diabetes.

Lower your saturated fat intake

We know that people who develop type 2 diabetes are more likely to have a high saturated fat intake. Saturated fat may promote insulin resistance, making it harder for insulin to do its job of regulating your blood glucose levels. To eat less saturated fat:

Use lower fat dairy products—Routinely purchase lower fat milk, cheese, custard, ice cream and yogurt rather than their regular forms.

Choose your snack foods wisely—Don't buy chocolates, cookies, potato chips, muffin bars, etc. See Chapter 13 for healthy snack options.

Cook with the good oils—The healthier oils to use are olive, canola and other seed and nut oils.

Take care when you are eating away from home—Give up the french fries and potato wedges with sour cream, along with other deep-fried foods and pizza.

Eat lean meats.

Boost your omega-3 intake

While high saturated fat intakes are associated with diabetes, there is one type of fat that's protective—the very long-chain omega-3 fatty acids. Dietary trials in animals and people have shown that increased omega-3 intake can improve insulin sensitivity and therefore could reduce diabetes risk.

Our bodies only make small amounts of these unique fatty acids, so we rely on dietary sources, especially fish and seafood, for them. Aim to include fish in your diet at least twice a week, such as a main meal of fresh fish *not* cooked in saturated fat, plus at least one sandwich-sized serving of, say, canned salmon or tuna.

> ### Which fish is best?
>
> **Oily fish,** which tend to have darker-colored flesh and a stronger flavor, are the richest source of omega-3 fats. Some examples are: herring, Atlantic salmon, smoked salmon, tuna, mackerel and sardines. Medium sources are: wild salmon, wild swordfish, rainbow trout, mussels, snapper, grouper, calamari, mackerel, oysters.
>
> **Canned fish** such as salmon, sardines, mackerel and, to a lesser extent, tuna are all good sources of omega-3s; look for canned fish packed in water, or brine—and drain the fish well.

As well as eating these great sources of long-chain omega-3s, you can also increase your total omega-3 intake by eating short-chain omega-3s, which are found in canola oil and margarine, nuts and seeds (particularly walnuts and flaxseeds), and legumes such as baked beans and soybeans.

Lower the GI of your diet

Studies show that people who base their diet on carbohydrates with a low GI are the least likely to develop type 2 diabetes. Some studies have suggested that simply changing the bread you eat can make a difference. Here are some key ways to lower the GI of your diet:

- Choose low GI breads such as grainy bread, authentic sourdough, soy and flaxseed bread or a fruit bread
- Swap high GI cereals such as corn flakes and puffed rice for less processed and higher fiber cereals such as rolled oats, traditional (not instant) oatmeal and natural muesli
- Limit cookies and bakery products and include fruit and lower fat milk or yogurt as low GI snacks
- Replace potato with sweet potato and corn, and

- Include legumes (home-cooked or canned beans, chickpeas and lentils) in your diet regularly.

Increase your fiber intake

Higher fiber intakes are also associated with a lower risk of type 2 diabetes. Specifically, higher intakes of wholegrain cereals and fruit and vegetables are recommended.

Get the benefit of whole grains (grains that are eaten in nature's packaging or close to it) with foods such as:

- Barley—try pearl barley in soup, or in recipes such as barley risotto or a barley salad
- Whole wheat or cracked wheat such as bulgur in tabouli
- Rolled oats or muesli for breakfast, and
- Wholegrain breads—the ones with chewy grains and seeds (low GI versions are best).

If you don't eat much fruit or vegetables at the moment, aim for at least one piece of fruit and two servings of vegetables each day. Build up gradually by eating one extra piece of fruit and one extra serving of vegetables each week.

If you are already eating quite a bit of fruit and vegetables, increase your intake until you reach two servings of fruit and five servings of vegetables every day.

Get regular physical activity

All the studies that have proven that a healthy lifestyle can prevent the development of type 2 diabetes have included a comprehensive exercise program in their definition of a healthy lifestyle. You need 150–300 minutes of moderate level physical activity each week, which is of course at least 30 minutes of activity each day. The kinds of activities that proved most useful to people with prediabetes included walking, jogging, cycling, swimming, dancing and ball games.

Chapter 22
Prediabetes:
Your daily food guide

With prediabetes the aim is to optimize your nutritional intake to minimize your risk of progression to diabetes and development of cardio-vascular disease. On average*, your daily food intake should include the following foods.

Your daily food guide

- 5–6 servings breads, cereals and other starchy foods
- 2–3 servings fruit
- 2–3 servings milk products or alternatives
- 2–3 servings meat or vegetarian alternatives
- 2–3 servings fat-rich foods, and
- 5 or more servings vegetables.

* The daily food guide is based on the requirements of a 50–60-year-old, overweight adult who is otherwise well and active in all normal daily activities. The calorie content is in the range of 1,400–2,000, with approximately 45 to 50 percent of energy from carbohydrate. Serving sizes can be found on pages 152 and 153.

How do you fit this into a day?

To illustrate what this looks like in terms of actual foods, we've laid out a meal plan showing the recommended number of servings distributed over the meals of a day. Beverages are not included unless they make a significant nutrient contribution.

Meal plan for an adult with prediabetes	Daily food servings	Example	Other ideas
Breakfast	1 serving bread, cereal or other starchy foods	⅓ cup crunchy muesli	toast, raisin toast, oatmeal or low GI breakfast cereal
	1 serving fruit	1 large fresh peach, diced	fruit, fresh or canned, juice or dried fruit
	1 serving milk product	1 cup fruit yogurt	milk on cereal or to drink
Lunch	2 servings bread	2 slices wholegrain bread	a bread roll, toast, wholegrain crackers, pasta, noodles
	2 servings vegetables	1 sliced tomato, ½ cucumber, 3 slices of beets and grated carrot	salad veggies or soup are good ways to boost intake
	1 serving meat or alternative	about 80g lean cooked roast beef	tuna, salmon, egg, mixed beans
	1 serving fat	1 tbsp mayonnaise on the sandwich	margarine, nut spreads, avocado or salad dressing
	1 serving milk product	1 glass lower fat milk	yogurt or other dairy dessert

Meal plan for an adult with prediabetes	Daily food servings	Example	Other ideas
Dinner	2 servings bread or other starchy food and 1 serving fat	1 potato and ¾ cup sweet potato baked with a little olive oil	rice, pasta or bread
	3 servings vegetables	baked pumpkin, beans, peas and broccoli	at least 1½ cups non-starchy vegetables
	1 serving meat or alternative	1 small drumstick and thigh of roast chicken (skin removed)	this protein component needs to be lean to keep saturated fat intake down
	1 serving fruit	1 cup fresh fruit salad	fruit salad, dried fruit or a small juice

MANAGING TYPE 2 DIABETES

If you have type 2 diabetes, your insulin does not work properly (insulin resistance) and/or you have a shortage of insulin. The aim of treatment is to help you make the best use of the insulin you have and to try to make it last as long as possible.

As we said in the introduction to this book, the most important thing you can do is to take control of your condition: get informed about what having diabetes means and what is recommended to manage diabetes and your health.

Because lifestyle factors contribute to type 2 diabetes, looking at the way you live (especially your diet and exercise habits) is the key to managing diabetes well.

Chapter 23
Living with type 2 diabetes

For some people with type 2 diabetes, all they have to do to keep their blood glucose levels in the normal range is manage their weight, eat a healthy diet and be active. Others also need to take pills, and some may need insulin.

The first thing you have to come to terms with when diagnosed with diabetes is that high blood glucose levels are probably not your only problem: you may also have high blood pressure, abnormal blood fats (high LDL (bad) cholesterol, low HDL (good) cholesterol and high triglycerides) and abdominal obesity (fat around the middle of your body). This is a potentially lethal health cocktail that increases your risk of developing major blood vessel diseases, especially heart disease, stroke and peripheral vascular disease (thrombosis), particularly of the lower limbs.

Second, it's highly likely that the way you have been living (diet and lack of exercise) contributed to your getting diabetes. So the first step for the majority of people with type 2 diabetes involves taking a good hard look at themselves and thinking about the changes they can make that will improve their blood glucose levels and blood fats and blood pressure, if they are higher than recommended.

For most people, the place to start is with what they eat.

You are what you eat

What changes do you need to make to your diet? Of course it varies, but these are the aspects for most people to focus on:

- **Reduce how much you eat.** Key foods to reduce are those high in saturated fats and/or added sugars, and alcohol. This doesn't mean just downsizing your daily chocolate bar from king size to standard (although this would definitely help). It means saving the chocolate bar for very special occasions only.

- **Cut back on saturated fats and cholesterol.** This is absolutely essential for everyone with type 2 diabetes. You must get and keep your LDL (bad) cholesterol down. Don't obsessively avoid high cholesterol eggs and prawns. It's the saturated fats in those lamb chops and chocolate chip cookies that are having the greatest effect on your cholesterol levels. If you've been eating healthily and doing regular exercise for at least three months and your cholesterol levels still haven't improved, talk to your doctor about cholesterol-lowering medications. A practical intermediate step may be to try one of the reduced fat margarines that have added phytosterols for a further three months. Provided you can eat the 4–5 teaspoons a day of margarine without gaining weight, these margarines can reduce your blood cholesterol levels by around 10 percent.

- **Modify your carbohydrate intake.** This means thinking about carb quality and quantity and getting familiar with the sources and amounts of carbohydrate in your diet. There's no point buying the "99 percent fat free" product if it packs in 120g of high GI carbs per serving. For carb quality, make sure that you are eating the low GI ones as much as possible. As for quantity, 30–60g of carbohydrate at any one sitting is an average range. Replacing some carbohydrate in your diet with monounsaturated fat can reduce your post-meal blood glucose levels and lower your triglycerides, but you have to be careful with this. Too much added fat may lead to weight gain. Talk to your dietitian about the proportion of fat to carbohydrate that's right for you.

- **Eat more regularly.** Whether you want to eat three meals a day or small meals plus snacks is up to you. However, if you use insulin or take medication that stimulates insulin production from your pancreas, it will be helpful if you can maintain some consistency in the times you eat your meals and the amount of carbohydrate you eat at those meals. A regimen of multiple insulin injections or use of a pump gives you more flexibility in your food intake.

- **Moderate your protein intake.** Protein won't increase your blood glucose level and is valuable for satisfying appetite. The usual recommended protein intake is 15–25 percent of your total energy intake. There is no need to eat any more.

- **Eat more of the healthy foods (such as fruit and vegetables).** You see, it isn't all about cutting back. Most people don't eat anywhere near enough of these foods. Fresh, dried and canned fruits are all suitable, and you can eat as much as you like of most non-starchy vegetables (leafy greens, carrots, tomatoes, onions, etc).

- **Cut back on salt.** Chances are you've got high blood pressure too. Reducing your sodium intake by not adding salt to food when cooking or at the table, and choosing salt reduced or low salt foods at the supermarket, is a great start. If you think you have done this but your blood pressure is still high, you might need medication as well. See your doctor for further advice.

Your healthy type 2 diabetes diet checklist

- Use poly and/or monounsaturated margarines and spreads instead of butter and butter blends.
- Use olive and/or canola oils in cooking and for salads.
- Don't drink more than 1–2 standard alcoholic drinks a day.
- Eat more than 3 cups (300g) of vegetables every day (this includes soups).
- Eat more than 2 pieces (200g) of fruit every day.
- Include legumes (canned or dried peas, beans or lentils) in your diet at least twice a week.
- Eat fish (100g or more) at least twice a week.
- Include lower fat dairy products (or calcium-enriched alternatives) in your diet daily and generally avoid full cream types.
- Eat wholegrain and high fiber cereals, breads and grains daily—look for the low GI ones.
- Eat lean red meat or poultry in moderately sized portions regularly.
- Drink 6–8 glasses of water, or other low calorie beverages, every day. Drinking more water won't lower your blood glucose levels, but high blood glucose means you should drink more water to avoid dehydration.

Did you know that as you age, you are at greater risk of dehydration as your sensitivity to thirst and your kidney function decline?

Exercise

The other aspect of your lifestyle to modify is exercise—because lack of it may have contributed to your getting diabetes. How much? You need to do at least 30–45 minutes, 3–5 days a week, or accumulate at least 150 minutes (that's 2½ hours) of exercise per week. And here's the pay-off for that 2½ hours exercise a week. It will:

- Improve your blood glucose levels
- Decrease your insulin resistance, and
- Reduce your risk of heart and blood vessel disease—which is the number one cause of death in people with diabetes.

What sort of exercise? The most beneficial forms of exercise are aerobic (walking) and resistance (weight lifting) exercise. Now before you scoff at the image of a geriatric Mr. or Mrs. Bodybuilder, you would be wise to heed the fact that older muscles are just as responsive to strength training as younger muscles. If you don't do something to maintain your muscles, they will shrink as you age. In fact a decrease in lean muscle mass and increase in body fat is the most common nutritional scenario in older people. It is never too late to get a set of light dumbbells and start training. Talk to your exercise specialist about a program that will suit you, not strain you.

For elderly people, one of the most important benefits of exercise is that it helps you stay mobile and independent. It will reduce the muscle wastage and frailty that make it difficult for you to care for yourself. You can rebuild weakened muscles and improve your balance to reduce the risk of falls and fractures. Exercise can even help maintain mental sharpness. Studies have shown that physical training improves mental function in elderly people with dementia.

Finally, it's worth noting that exercise can be a valuable mood enhancer in times of stress. People who are physically active are far less likely to be depressed, tense, confused, anxious and stressed out.

Any possibility of pregnancy?

If you're a woman with type 2 diabetes, and you're planning a pregnancy (or even if you're not planning it), you ought to talk to a doctor about what you need to do *before* you become pregnant (or talk about contraception). It is essential that your blood glucose levels are well managed before conception, to reduce the chance of miscarriage, deformities and other complications. A dietary supplement of folate (5 mg per day) is also recommended, and your doctor may want you to stop or change your diabetes medications. So make sure you see your doctor before you conceive for a complete diabetes health review (see also Chapter 31).

Q&A

Why is my blood glucose level higher in the morning than when I go to bed at night? I swear I don't eat anything during the night.

A higher blood glucose level (above 108 mg/dL) when you get up in the morning is a very common feature of type 2 diabetes and, understandably, a puzzle to many who experience it.

Part of the reason for it is what's described as the "dawn phenomenon." This is a normal physiological process: certain hormones in your body set to work to raise your blood glucose levels before you wake up. The hormones stimulate glucose production and release from your liver and inhibit glucose use by your body. The result is an increase in your blood glucose levels, ensuring that you have a supply of fuel ready for your wakening body's needs.

Other possible causes are more likely if you are taking insulin. If the insulin you took at night is running out by the morning, this could mean your blood glucose levels will be high when you wake up.

Are there any foods I can eat to improve my cholesterol levels?

Foods that will improve your cholesterol levels by lowering the bad (LDL) cholesterol and raising the good (HDL) cholesterol include those rich in polyunsaturated and monounsaturated oils (sunflower, safflower, canola and olive, nuts and seeds), plant sterol-enriched margarines, soy protein (soy beverages, tofu, soybeans) and foods that are low GI and high in soluble fiber.

Foods high in soluble fiber include legumes (lentils, peas and beans), whole grains such as barley, oats, and fruits and vegetables. A recently published study has found that including a combination of these high fiber foods in your diet can be as effective at lowering LDL cholesterol as the new generation of cholesterol-lowering drugs known as statins (Lipitor, Zocor, Lipex, Simvar, Pravachol, Vastin, Lescol).

Some foods help your cholesterol profile by raising levels of the HDL cholesterol. Omega-3 fatty acids—found in fish, soybean oil, avocados and walnuts—raise HDL levels and even have blood-thinning and antiarrhythmic properties that help maintain normal heart rhythm and reduce your risk of heart problems.

Some studies have shown that moderate consumption of alcohol (1–2 drinks per day) also leads to increased levels of HDL. However, because of the other health risks associated with alcohol consumption, doctors recommend that non-drinkers don't start drinking.

Some experts suspect that high blood levels of the amino acid homocysteine promote atherosclerosis (hardening and narrowing of the arteries). Increasing your intake of folic acid, vitamin B6 and vitamin B12 can help reduce levels of homocysteine. Natural sources of these vitamins include leafy greens, legumes, whole grains, lean meats and nuts.

I've heard that coffee is good for diabetes. Is that true?

There are studies both for and against coffee in relation to diabetes. Occasional coffee drinking may actually decrease insulin sensitivity, but drinking coffee or other high caffeine foods or beverages on a regular basis does not appear to have any detrimental effects on people with diabetes in the long run. The body seems to adapt to the caffeine so that it no longer has any negative effects.

Coffee (regular and decaffeinated) contains lots of antioxidants and magnesium, which may improve insulin sensitivity. A study of the dietary habits of more than 125,000 people in the US over 20 years found that men who drank more than six cups of caffeinated coffee a day reduced their chances of getting type 2 diabetes by more than 50 percent compared with men in the study who didn't drink coffee.

Among the women, those who drank six or more cups a day reduced their risk of type 2 diabetes by nearly 30 percent. These effects could not be accounted for by lifestyle factors such as smoking, exercise or obesity. Decaffeinated coffee was also beneficial, but it had less effect than regular coffee.

Chapter 24
Type 2 diabetes: Your daily food guide

As an adult with type 2 diabetes, you have similar nutritional requirements to someone without diabetes, but meeting those requirements should take on a higher priority for you now. On average*, your daily food intake should include the following foods:

Your daily food guide

- 5–6 servings breads and cereals and other starchy foods
- 2–3 servings fruits
- 2–3 servings of milk products or alternatives
- 1–2 servings meat or vegetarian alternatives
- 2–3 servings fat-rich foods, and
- 5 or more servings vegetables.

*The daily food guide is based on a 60-year-old, overweight adult who is active in usual daily living. The calorie content will range from 1,300–1,900 with approximately 50 percent energy from carbohydrates. Serving sizes can be found on pages 152 and 153.

How do you fit this into a day?

Here's an example of how you could fit this food into a day. Beverages are not included except where they make a significant nutrient contribution.

Meal plan for an adult with type 2 diabetes	Daily food servings	Example	Other ideas
Breakfast	1 serving bread, cereal or other starchy food with ½ serving fats	1 slice flaxseed toast spread with margarine	toast, oatmeal, muesli, rice
	1 serving fruit	topped with sliced banana	a glass of juice, a tablespoon of raisins, an apple
	1 serving milk products	and a coffee with skim milk	milk or yogurt on cereal, or a glass of milk to drink
Lunch	2 servings bread, cereal or other starchy food	a seeded bread roll	rice, pasta, potato, or bread
	2 servings vegetables	a handful of lettuce, 1 sliced tomato, ½ small cucumber and 2 sliced mushrooms	any combination of vegetables or salad
	1 serving fat-rich food	¼ avocado	margarine, mayonnaise or even a handful of nuts
	1 serving fruit	2 large fresh apricots	any piece of fresh fruit, a bowl of fruit salad, or a cup of canned fruit

Meal plan for an adult with type 2 diabetes	Daily food servings	Example	Other ideas
Dinner	2 servings other starchy foods and ½ serving fat-rich food	1 small sweet potato with a teaspoon of margarine	noodles, rice, sweetcorn, lentils
	1 serving meat or alternative	100g beef steak	fish, cheese, chicken, tofu
	3 servings vegetables	1½ cups steamed seasonal vegetables dressed with a teaspoon of lemon juice	3 cups of salad vegetables
	1 serving milk products	7 ounces lite peach and passionfruit yogurt	a cup of cocoa, a carton of yogurt or some ice cream

Chapter 25
Type 2 diabetes in children

In the past, when a child was diagnosed with diabetes, the typical symptoms of weight loss, dehydration and thirst made it easy to classify as type 1, juvenile onset or insulin-dependent diabetes. In recent years a new picture has emerged:

- Instead of being thin, this child is fat, and
- Instead of the body not making insulin, the body is making lots of insulin.

If you are a young person with type 2 diabetes (or if you have a child with type 2), this chapter will tell you what to do about it.

And if you have type 2 diabetes, your children are also at risk of this disease; this chapter will also show you the types of diet and lifestyle changes which will reduce their risk.

Young people with diabetes — a new epidemic

There is currently no cure for diabetes. It's for life. Not only that, but children with type 2 diabetes face the same risk of complications as adults with type 2—heart attack, stroke, impotence, blindness, kidney disease. But not when they are old or retired. Children who develop type 2 diabetes will be facing these health problems at the peak of their adult life, when their working and earning capacity is greatest and when they have their own young families to educate and care for. For the individual, the implications are terrible; for the public health system, the burden is overwhelming.

For obese children and teenagers, the diagnosis of type 2 diabetes is really just the final straw because their fatness has an impact on them every day of their lives. It's no fun being fat in a world that equates attractiveness and intelligence with body shape. Maintaining high self-esteem can be very difficult for fat children. Just getting through each day is of much greater concern to them than the high blood pressure, orthopedic problems and high blood fats that commonly precede the diagnosis of type 2 diabetes.

**Obese children, in particular older children,
are very likely to become obese adults.**

How is it diagnosed?

Type 2 diabetes in young people, just as in adults, usually develops over several years, and there may not be any easily recognizable symptoms. Children with type 2 diabetes are usually overweight or obese and have a strong family history of type 2 diabetes. There are a couple of things to watch for:

- They are very likely to have Acanthosis nigricans, a dark pigmentation of the skin around the neck, which is a marker of insulin resistance, and
- Girls are also more likely to have polycystic ovarian syndrome (PCOS).

Just about all the symptoms indicative of type 1 diabetes can occur in a child with type 2 diabetes so diagnosis can be difficult. Blood tests confirming the absence of antibodies against the insulin-producing cells are necessary.

How is it treated?

Managing type 2 in kids is a family affair, and there are some (possibly major) diet and lifestyle changes the whole family is going to have to make. The good news is that these changes are good for everyone's health and wellbeing.

Who is responsible for what?

- Parents are responsible for choosing *when*, *where* and *what* is available to eat, and
- Children are responsible for choosing *how much* and *even whether* they eat.

Type 2 diabetes can be managed successfully through a combination of regular physical activity, healthy eating and, for some young people, medication, including insulin. The aim is to:
- Normalize blood glucose levels
- Reduce blood fats (cholesterol and triglycerides) and blood pressure, and
- Prevent the progression or development of complications.

One of the key ways to achieve these goals is by managing weight: intake of energy from food has to decrease, and output of energy (physical activity) has to increase.

Whether or not medication is needed depends on how high the blood glucose levels are—particularly when first diagnosed. Insulin injections are usually the first choice because most of the oral blood glucose-lowering medications have not yet been properly tested in young people. However, metformin is prescribed in some countries, along with insulin. Once the blood glucose levels have come down, the young person may be able to come off insulin.

Physical activity

Increasing energy output through physical activity is absolutely essential to managing type 2 diabetes—in adults and children. If you want to see results in terms of fat loss, extra physical activity will bring about improvements more quickly than diet alone, making it a great motivational tool. Also, regular exercise can improve self-esteem and reduce depression and anxiety.

Just like for adults with type 2 diabetes, a minimum of 30 minutes of some kind of physical activity, most days of the week, is essential for children. At least double that to lose weight!

Parents: when looking at your lifestyle, think about how you can reduce sedentary behavior and increase planned and incidental activity for everybody.

Family business—how the whole family can get moving and eat better

Limit screen time

Did you know that 5 hours a week sitting passively instead of moving amounts to more than 2 lbs of body fat not burned off every month? In most families, getting kids to be more active usually starts with limiting screen time—TV, computers, iPads, smart phones, PlayStations, movies, etc.

An Australian study found that children who watched TV for more than 2 hours per day were more likely to consume high energy snacks and drinks and less likely to participate in organized sports.

**If you want to get your kids more active,
you have to be more active yourself.**

Activate your child's day

Parental activity is a strong predictor of a child's activity, so start by taking a long hard look at your own lifestyle and figuring out how you could all move a bit more.

It's not hard to increase incidental activity. Get the whole family involved in helping with household tasks (including setting and clearing the table, doing the dishes, making their own beds, cleaning rooms and ironing their own clothes once they are old enough), and family activities (including shopping, sweeping the yard, mowing the lawn and walking the dog).

Planned activity can mean participating in organized sports such as tennis, basketball, football, hockey, track, T-ball, baseball, gymnastics, etc. If your children are not really into organized sports and prefer something individual that they can do at their own pace, there are plenty of other options, such as riding a bike, going for a swim, going for a walk, dancing or a martial art.

Whatever they choose, make sure they enjoy it. If they don't, try something else.

A healthier family diet

There are many approaches to managing the diet of a child with type 2 diabetes. They range from weighed and measured calorie controlled plans to guided, progressive habit changes such as eating more fruit and limiting the number of treat foods. We suggest you and your child see an accredited dietitian to discuss and plan the right approach for you—this needs to be someone you are both comfortable talking to and working with over the long haul.

Whatever you do, it helps if the whole family eats the same way. This way you are all in it together, and the child with diabetes is supported. Also, it makes meal preparation much easier. The whole family will benefit in terms of health and fitness. What's more, it's very likely that someone else in the family has diabetes too.

The daily food guide in Chapter 26 will give you an idea of what's involved and how to get started.

Quick-fix weight loss plans are not a good idea for children because of children's nutritional requirements and because type 2 diabetes is a lifelong condition.

Five of the best

Here are five proven strategies for achieving a healthier household diet:

- Have regular family meals
- Serve a variety of healthy foods and snacks
- Be a good role model by eating healthily yourself
- Involve kids in the process of food choice and preparation, and
- Avoid battles over food.

Have regular family meals

Family meals are a comforting ritual for children and a great way to end the day. Children like the routine, and parents get a chance to catch up with what's been going on in everyone's lives. Research suggests other benefits too. Children who take part in regular family meals are also:

- More likely to eat fruits, vegetables and whole grains
- Less likely to snack on unhealthy foods, and
- Less likely to smoke, use marijuana or drink alcohol.

Independent teenagers may turn up their noses at the prospect of a family meal. But despite what they say, they often do value parental guidance (not interference), so use meal times as a chance to reconnect in a relaxed way. Get to know their friends by inviting them over to dinner, too. Or get some help in the kitchen by involving them in planning and preparation.

What counts as a family meal? Any time you and your family sit down around the table and eat together—whether it's take-out food or a home-cooked meal. Maybe this means you have to eat a little later because you wait until someone gets home from work, or perhaps you set aside breakfast on the weekend as a leisurely family affair. Whenever it is, strive for healthy food (deliciously prepared, of course) and a happy, harmonious atmosphere (without TV).

Serve a variety of healthy foods and snacks

Children, especially younger ones, eat mostly what you have in the pantry, fridge and freezer. That's why it's important (and relatively easy) to control the supply lines—the foods that you serve for meals and have on hand for snacks. Here are some basic guidelines:

- Limit drinks such as fruit juice and soft drinks to once a day: offer water and plain, lower fat milk instead

- Include a low GI food with each meal: studies have shown this can have a profound effect on lowering both fasting and overall 24-hour glucose profiles
- Don't put any limits on fruits and vegetables: instead, work on including some at each meal and snack
- Make eating fresh fruit easy by washing, peeling or slicing and presenting it attractively without any competition (like cookies)
- Serve lean meats, fish and poultry rather than sausages and chicken nuggets and include other good sources of protein, such as eggs and nuts
- Limit fat intake by using lower fat dairy products and avoiding deep-fried foods, and
- Avoid packaged snacks (chips, crackers, cereal and muffin bars) as much as possible: low-fat varieties are not filling and not a good alternative. But don't completely ban your children's favorite snacks— make them one of the "keep for a treat" foods.

What's a treat food? It's a food kept for a very special occasion. It's not an every day or even every second day food. Perhaps once a week?

Snacks

Children need regular meals and snacks (around 5–6 occasions of eating per day). Young children generally can't meet their energy needs for growth and activity with just three meals. For older children, snacks make up half to a third of their energy intake, so it is important that the snacks you offer contribute as much in terms of nutrients as they do in energy.

If they are on the go or if you find portion control helpful, pre-packaged single serving snacks can be useful. Muesli bars, drinking yogurts, yogurt and muesli mixes, nut bars, dried fruit and nut mixes, dried fruit bars, packs of cheese slices all fall into this category. But if it comes prepackaged, read the label carefully and compare brands. Here are some ideas for healthy, portable snacks:

- A lower fat flavored milk
- A muesli bar
- Fresh fruit, cut up
- Lower fat yogurt
- Handfuls of raw vegetables—carrot sticks, fresh green beans, celery pieces, cucumber, mini tomatoes, bell pepper strips
- A matchbox-sized piece of cheese
- A handful of dried apple rings
- A small bottle of drinking yogurt
- A cup of vegetable or pumpkin soup with toast fingers
- A slice of fruit toast
- A small carton of fruit salad
- Breakfast cereal and lower fat milk
- A handful of dried apricots, raisins and almonds, and
- Wholegrain crackers with spread.

Why snack?

- Because of hunger
- To prevent lows and maintain their blood glucose levels between meals
- To pick up an extra serving of fruit or dairy
- To lower the glycemic load of their main meals (by reducing their size)
- To prevent excessive hunger and subsequent overindulgence, and
- To overcome a mid-afternoon slump in energy levels.

Be a good role model by eating healthily yourself

Dieting is a not a normal way of eating. If you have a controlling and restrictive approach to food, try not to pass it on to your children; get some help yourself. Here's what you should do:

- Eat the foods you would like your children to eat, and
- Don't classify foods as "good" or "bad" or forbid certain foods.

Instead, teach your kids that all foods can be eaten—some every day, others sometimes. Avoid using food, for example dessert, as a reward.

Withholding a child's favorite food can make him or her feel powerless and is likely to increase his or her desire for it.

Children have an excellent built-in ability to sense when they are full, so pushing them to eat everything on their plate with the temptation of a treat afterward can actually condition them to overeat.

Involve kids in the process of food choice and preparation

Teach them how to cook. Grow some vegetables: little cherry tomatoes, strawberries or lettuce can easily be grown in pots, and they taste delicious. Take them to a farm or orchard when it's picking season. Let them select a new fruit or vegetable to try in the grocery store. Have them shop for food with you (sometimes). Get to know local shopkeepers—at the butcher's or fruit market, bakery or deli. If you're a regular, many will be only too pleased to give a little one a taste of something.

Avoid battles over food

Children are naturally "neophobic"—which means being afraid of new things—so it is normal for them to refuse new foods. Vegetables included! Some people believe this is a protective instinct, but it can be excruciatingly frustrating to parents.

You can work on overcoming this tendency by exposing them often to whatever is the new food, so that pretty soon it is no longer new and unfamiliar. You have to be persistent. Offer a new food 5 to 10 times in small amounts, without pressuring your child to eat it, and gradually you should see some acceptance. Praise any efforts at tasting new foods.

Give their tastebuds time to adjust

Making gradual changes is more successful than making extreme changes overnight. Children's taste for fat, for instance, will diminish as you decrease the amount of fat in their food.

It takes about six weeks for children's tastebuds to adapt to new tastes, so give them time.

For example, after a few months on low-fat milk, they'll find whole milk way too creamy—it will be too rich for their new palate.

Chapter 26
Daily food guide for children with type 2 diabetes

Good nutrition is essential in youth to optimize growth and development. With type 2 diabetes there is the added need to aim for a diet that minimizes the risk of progression or development of complications like blood vessel disease. On average* the daily diet should include something along these lines:

Your daily food guide

- 8–12 servings breads, cereals and other starchy foods
- 2–4 servings fruit
- 2–3 servings milk products or alternatives
- 2 servings meat or vegetarian alternatives
- 2–4 servings fat-rich foods, and
- 5 or more servings vegetables.

*The daily food guide is designed to meet the nutrient requirements of an overweight teenager (14–18 years) who is active in all daily living and does some regular moderate exercise. It provides 1,550–2,000 calories with approximately 50 percent energy coming from carbohydrate. Serving sizes can be found on pages 152 and 153.

How do you fit this into a day?

Here is an example of how these daily food needs can fit into a day.

Meal plan for a young person with type 2 diabetes	Daily food servings	Example	Other ideas
Breakfast	4 servings bread, cereal or other starchy food and 2 fat sources	4 slices grain toast with margarine	home-made hot cakes or muffins
	1 serving fruit	a small orange juice	fresh or dried fruit
	½ serving meat or alternative	2 slices processed cheese	an egg, lean bacon
Mid-morning	1 serving fruit	an apple	
Lunch	4 servings bread, cereal or other starchy food	2 slices toast and ¾ cup refried beans	bread, rolls, pasta, rice noodles
	1 serving vegetable plus 1 fat serving	½ cup coleslaw	cherry tomatoes, carrot sticks, cucumber
	1 serving milk product	a glass of low-fat milk	yogurt, flavored milk, dairy dessert
	½ serving meat or alternative	an omega-3 rich egg	ham, cheese, canned fish
Mid-afternoon	1 serving milk product	a carton of yogurt	milk, low-fat ice cream
	1 serving fruit	a small banana	

Meal plan for a young person with type 2 diabetes	Daily food servings	Example	Other ideas
Dinner	4 servings bread, cereal or other starchy food	1 ear of corn and 1 small sweet potato	legumes, pasta, rice
	1 serving meat or alternative	2–3 trimmed lamb cutlets	chicken, fish, lean minced beef
	4 servings vegetables	2 cups of mixed vegetables	any mixture of low-starch vegetables
	1 serving fruit	½ cup canned fruit	fresh fruit salad or frozen fruit

Chapter 27

Managing diabetes when eating out, on special occasions . . . and what about chocolate?

Eating out can really test your resolve as far as healthy eating goes. But, like most things, the more often you do it, the more important it is to get it right. If you only eat out once a month, there's no need to be too fussy with what you eat. But if it's three or four times a week, whether for business or pleasure, making good choices is critical to your nutritional wellbeing.

When we eat out we tend to eat more than we would at home. And in most places, we're likely to get a lot more salt, refined carbohydrate and fat than we would from home-cooked food. This chapter tells you the best menu choices for a wide range of cuisines and gives you tips for eating out at the movies, lunch bars, cafés, pubs, on a flight, and for fast food, including McDonald's and KFC.

The health guide to what's on the menu

Asian meals

Asian meals including Chinese, Thai, Indian and Japanese, offer a great variety of foods which you can put together to create a healthy meal.

Keeping in mind the three steps to a balanced meal, seek out a low GI carb such as low GI rice, dhal, sushi or noodles. Chinese and Thai traditionally use jasmine rice, and although it is usually high GI, a small serving of steamed rice is better for you than fried rice or fried noodles.

Adding some protein gives staying power—try marinated tofu, stir-fried seafood, tandoori chicken, sashimi tuna, fish tikka or lean beef. Be cautious with pork and duck—fattier cuts are often used—and avoid Thai curries and dishes made with coconut milk.

Remember, the third dish to order is steamed or stir-fried vegetables! Go easy on extras, especially the deep-fried ones—spring rolls, dim sims, pakoras and tempura. These are often served as an entrée, so they get you when your appetite is greatest. Don't order them if you can help it.

And remember, while someone's picking up the tandoori or teriyaki take-out, you can be stir-frying the vegetables at home. In a frypan or wok, heat a teaspoon of sesame oil and stir-fry 2 teaspoons crushed garlic, 1 tablespoon crushed ginger and 3 finely chopped shallots for 30 seconds. Add 5 cups sliced broccoli with the stalks trimmed (plus other Asian greens if you have them on hand) and ½ cup chicken stock. Cover and steam. Serve with soy sauce.

Good menu options include all the following:

Chinese

- Steamed dim sims or dumplings
- Clear soups containing noodles/wontons and vegetables
- Vegetable-based dishes such as chop suey

- Braised skinless chicken or beef dishes in chili, oyster, soy or garlic sauces
- Seafood dishes such as curried prawns, scallops with ginger and shallots, steamed whole fish
- Stir-fried or steamed vegetables, and
- Noodles or smaller servings of steamed or boiled rice.

Thai

- Fresh spring rolls
- Tom yum goong (hot and sour soup)—it's a good low calorie stomach filler
- Any Thai salad
- Noodles in soups rather than fried in pad thai
- Seafood braised in a sauce with vegetables
- Wok-tossed tofu (bean curd), seafood, chicken, beef, lamb or pork fillet with nuts, vegetables and sauce
- Smaller servings of steamed jasmine rice, and
- Stir-fried mixed vegetables with garlic and oyster sauce or Thai herbs.

Indian

- Unleavened bread such as chapatis, plain naan or roti
- Beef, chicken, seafood or vegetable curry
- Tikka (dry roasted) or tandoori (marinated in spices and yogurt) chicken, prawns or fish
- Basmati rice—a great lower GI accompaniment, but watch the quantity!
- Dhal—an even better accompaniment, being very low GI, and
- Vegetable dishes such as stir-fried vegetables, vegetable curry, channa (a delicious chickpea curry), spicy spinach (saag), fresh salad and side orders such as pickles, cucumber raita, tomato and onion.

Japanese

- Miso soup or the more substantial udon soup
- Sushi, with seafood, chicken or vegetable
- Teriyaki (grilled meat or seafood with a special sauce)
- Teppan yaki (chargrilled steak, seafood and veggies)
- Yakitori (skewered chicken and onions in teriyaki sauce)
- Sashimi (thinly sliced raw beef, salmon or tuna—a great way to stock up on omega-3 fats)
- Shabu-shabu (thin slices of beef quickly cooked with mushrooms, cabbage and other vegetables), and
- Side orders like seaweed salad, edamame (young green soybeans), wasabi (horseradish), shoyu (soy sauce) and oshinko (pickled ginger).

Mexican and Spanish

Mexican restaurants are ideal for low GI choices because they make such great use of beans. Many of the dishes are very high in carbohydrates, though, because they include rice and corn as well. Probably the biggest nutritional hazards are cheese—they use lots of it—and sour cream. You can ask for these to be served separately. They do some salads as accompaniments. Good menu options include:

- Bean and salsa dips (tomato-based rather than cheese-based)
- Gazpacho or black bean soup
- Salads with grilled chicken or lamb
- Seafood
- Shellfish paella (spicy rice with seafood, tomato and saffron)
- Enchiladas (corn tortillas filled with meat or cheese with chili sauce), and
- Burritos (filled flour tortillas) and fajitas.

Italian

You'll find lots of low GI pasta in an Italian restaurant, but it might be best to order an appetizer—it will be plenty big enough. Many pasta dishes also use a lot of cheese, so balance your meal by having a fresh salad with it. Steer clear of crumbed and deep-fried seafood and watch out for creamy sauces. Good menu options include:

- Minestrone, stracciatella (soups)
- Prosciutto (paper-thin slices of smoky ham) wrapped around melon
- Barbecued marinated seafood dishes
- Entrée-sized pasta with tomato (napolitana), bean (fagoli) or seafood (marinara) sauce (without cream)
- Cannelloni with ricotta and spinach
- Grilled fish
- Roast or chargrilled fillet of beef, lamb loin or poultry
- Green garden salad with olive oil and balsamic vinegar
- Tomato salads with basil, olive oil and lemon juice
- Vegetarian pizza, and
- Gelato or sorbet or a fresh fruit platter.

Greek and Middle Eastern

Mediterranean cuisine uses a lot of olive oil, lemon, garlic, onions and other vegetables. Many dishes are chargrilled—specialties such as barbecued octopus or grilled sardines are excellent choices. You'll find regular bread and potatoes replaced with flatbread and Turkish bread, and whole grains such as bulgur (cracked wheat) (in tabouli) and couscous (semolina pasta) in stuffed eggplant and capsicum. Good menu options include:

- Meze platter with pita bread. Among the small appetizing dishes here you could pick and choose what you like. There are healthy dips to enjoy in small quantities, such as hummus, baba ghanoush, tzatziki and taramasalata with tasty extras of olives and dolmades

- Souvlaki—chargrilled skewers of meat or chicken with vegetables
- Kofta or kibbi balls of minced lamb with bulgur (cracked wheat)
- Stifatho—a lamb, potato and onion casserole
- Greek salad of tomato, olives, feta cheese, capsicum, with balsamic dressing or oil and lemon (you could ask for the dressing on the side) or tabouli salad
- Cabbage rolls, stuffed tomatoes, and
- Fresh fruit platter.

How to hurdle nutritional hazards with fast food and take-out

You're out and about, on the go and there it is, that grumbling grouch in your belly—hunger pangs have hit! You need to eat and you need to eat now! So how good are you at finding something decent to eat in the big wide world of fast food?

Did you think you were bypassing the fat with a new-fashioned warm salad or freshly made roll? The truth is you might do just as well with a burger, but remember, a decent burger with all the extras and cheese has about 30g of fat and over 1100 mg of sodium. It probably shouldn't be your first choice if you're trying to lose weight and improve your ability to utilize insulin.

How do you decide what's good to eat when there's so much to choose from? If that angel inside you has been losing the argument in the "eat it" "don't eat it" battle lately, you probably owe it the courtesy of taking a look at this . . .

Café and pub food

Nutritional hazards	Better options
Beverages • Super-sized gourmet coffee and hot chocolate • Oversized juices • Regular soft drinks	**Beverages** • Skim or reduced fat milk coffees • Water, mineral water or regular-sized freshly squeezed fruit and vegetable juices • Diet soft drinks
Light meals • Buttery herb or garlic bread • Spring rolls and other deep-fried morsels • Ham and cheese croissants • Club sandwich	**Light meals** • Bruschetta (with tomato, basil, olive oil) • Soups (watch for cream or coconut milk) • Salads • BLTs (go light on the mayo) • Smoked salmon bagels
Mains • Chicken schnitzel • Beef and onion burger • Pasta carbonara • Large pasta with pesto and parmesan • Fried seafood basket • Nachos with corn chips, cheese and sour cream	**Mains** • Chargrilled steak or skinless chicken breast • Vegetable-topped pizza (thin crust) • Appetizer-sized pasta dishes with tomato-based sauce (such as bolognese, marinara, napolitana, arrabiata) • Seafood such as marinated calamari, grilled with chilis and lemon or steamed mussels with a tomato sauce

Nutritional hazards	Better options
Sides • Fries, wedges, mashed potato	**Sides** • Steamed vegetables or side salads
Breakfasts • Sausage, bacon • Croissants • Hash browns • Pastries	**Breakfasts** • Smoked salmon • Poached eggs • Raisin toast • Sourdough or wholegrain bread
Sweets • Baked cheesecake, caramel cake, brownies	**Sweets** • A single little cookie or a skim or reduced fat milk iced chocolate

At the movies

Nutritional hazards	Better options
• Anything beyond a small popcorn	• Small popcorn
• Anything beyond a 1.5 oz bag of potato chips, corn chips	• 1.5 oz bag of chips
• Brand-name ice creams	• Soft serve or choc top
• Big chocolate bars	• Go for something smaller

Lunch bars

Nutritional hazards	Better options
• White bread • Big bread like focaccia (unless you want lots of carbs)	• Mixed grain or sourdough bread • Avocado or hummus instead of margarine or butter

Nutritional hazards	Better options
• Salami, sausage fillings	• Salad fillings for sandwiches or as a side order instead of fries
• Cheese every day (a generous serving can add as much fat as fries)	• Tubs of fresh rice, bean, garden or Greek salad
• Fries, fries, fries	• Pasta dishes with a mixture of vegetables and meat
• Full fat milkshakes	• Lebanese kebabs with tabouli and hummus
• Anything deep-fried, including chicken schnitzel, fish cocktails, spring rolls, scallops	• Grilled fish rather than fried fish
• A burger with "everything"	• Vegetarian pizza
	• Gourmet wraps
	• Tubs of fruit salad
	• Burritos with beans, lettuce, tomato and a little cheese (skip the sour cream!)
	• Frozen yogurt or reduced or low-fat yogurt mixed with fresh fruits
	• A skinny smoothie

In-flight

Nutritional hazards	Better options
• White bread, cheese, salami, cake and pastries (in airport lounges)	• Fresh fruit, soup and salad
• Packaged cake or muffin, cheese and crackers, cookies, ice cream or chocolate bar (offered as a snack in flight)	• Dried fruit, nut bars, bananas or apples that you have brought yourself
• Too much alcohol	• Plenty of water

Fast food worlds

Fast food outlets do offer the advantage of having the nutritional composition of their menus available, so we took a closer look to see what we could recommend. Some of the options stood out as being either

- too high in fat, or
- too high in carbohydrate for most people.

  We've highlighted this with:

★ = more than 20g of fat/serving

❖ = more than 60g of carbohydrate/serving.

Wendy's

Nutritional hazards	Better options
Hamburgers	**Hamburgers**
• Dave's Hot'n Juicy ½ lb double or triple★	• Smaller burgers, e.g., Dave's ¼ lb single
• Baconator ★	• Chicken burgers and wraps
Salads	**Salads**
• Spicy Chicken Caesar salad full size★	• Half size salads or Asian Cashew Chicken Salad
	• Garden or Caesar side salads
Sides	**Sides**
• Large Natural Cut Fries❖	• Sour cream & chives or Cheese & Broccoli Baked Potato❖
	• Apple slices
Beverages	**Beverages**
• Large sodas❖	• Diet sodas or water
• Frostys❖	• Jr Frosty

KFC

Nutritional hazards	Better options
Chicken	**Chicken**
• Multiple pieces of fried chicken	• Individual pieces of chicken, especially Kentucky Grilled Chicken or Extra Crispy Tenders
Extras	**Extras**
• KFC Famous Bowls— Mashed Potato with Gravy★❖	• Snack sized bowl of Mashed Potato with Gravy
• Chicken Pot Pie★❖	• Green beans, mashed potato, corn on the cob, BBQ Baked beans, coleslaw, Sweet kernel corn, KFC Cornbread Muffins
• Chicken Littles	
• Hot Wings	
• Go Cups	
Beverages	**Beverages**
• Anything above a 16 oz regular soda❖	• Diet sodas or small servings

Burger King

Nutritional hazards	Better options
Hamburgers	**Hamburgers**
• Whopper Sandwich with Cheese★	• Whopper Jr. Sandwich
• Double Whopper Sandwich★	• Flame Broiled Burgers
• Double Whopper Sandwich with Cheese★	• Tendergrill Chicken Sandwich
• Triple Whopper★	• Big Fish Sandwich
• Four Cheese Whopper★	• BK Veggie Burger
Salads and Sides	**Salads and Sides**
• Tendercrisp chicken	• Chicken and salad wraps
• Large fries❖	• Tendergrill salads

Nutritional hazards	Better options
Breakfast	**Breakfast**
• BK Ultimate Breakfast Platter★❖	• Quaker Oatmeal
• Double Croissan'wich w/ Sausage, Egg and Cheese★	• BK Breakfast Muffin Sandwich
• Sausage or Bacon Egg and Cheese Biscuit★	
Beverages	**Beverages**
• Shakes❖, especially bigger than 12 oz★❖	• 12oz Smoothies
• 20 oz and above sodas, Fruit Punch, Frappes	• Diet sodas, unsweetened tea, Light lemonade, small Lattes or hot chocolate

Taco Bell

Nutritional hazards	Better options
Meal items	**Meal items**
• XXL Grilled Stuft Burrito❖	• Chalupas
• Beefy Fritos Burrito	• Fresco Burritos and soft tacos
• Beefy 5-layer, Seven Layer Burrito	• Gordita Supreme
• Cheesy Potato Burrito	
• Nachos BellGrande❖	
Sides & Specialities	• Black Beans, Black Beans & Rice
• Smothered Burritos❖	
• Quesarito❖	• Mini Quesadillas
• Taco Salads❖	• Tostadas
Beverages	**Beverages**
• Large Freezes❖	• Brisk Iced Tea and Lemonade
• Large soda drinks	• Coffee
	• Diet sodas
	• SoBe Lifewater Yumberry Pomegranate

On the road

Traveling away from home means stepping out of your routine—it can be harder to eat well, and much, much easier to miss meals. Here are a few tips about what to take:

- Tuna and salmon in foil pouches (remember to pack a plastic fork)
- Salt reduced instant packet soups (all you need is boiling water and a mug)
- Ryvita
- Dried apricots, apples, etc.
- Dried fruit bars, and
- Portion-controlled packs of unsalted nuts or dried fruit.

Special occasions

Christmas, birthdays, entertaining, celebrations, parties—all these events have one thing in common: food! The circumstances might present some challenges:

- The foods served may be new to you, so you won't be sure how to fit them into your diet
- The time of meals may be different from your usual schedule
- The amount of food may be more or less than you usually eat, and
- Special occasions are also occasions for treat foods—chocolate features in a big way at Christmas and especially Easter.

So what do you do? Kick back and let your hair down? Or hide away and avoid life? There is a middle path—you don't want to knock yourself around, but you want to have a good time too. If you want to feel good after your next special occasion, try taking a positive approach to doing things a bit differently.

10 tips to successful socializing

- Don't arrive hungry: if you have a small healthy snack before you leave home, you'll reduce the chance that you'll overeat when you get to the party.

- Don't stockpile your plate with treats you don't need: if it's a buffet, take one or two items and only come back for more if you genuinely need to.

- Smaller portions can help you stay in control: try eating a small amount of several foods. This way you can eat what you like.

- Adopt a pastry-free policy: if you avoid these calorie-laden party foods, you'll be ahead.

- Talk more, eat less, and move away from the food table.

- Take to the dance floor to burn up some or all the excess energy.

- Alternate alcoholic and non-alcoholic drinks.

- Use small wine glasses: a standard glass of wine is 3½ ounces, not the 10 ounces the latest and largest glasses can hold (incidentally, they aren't meant to be filled to the brim).

- Fill your glass yourself, and only when it's empty: it's very easy to lose count of top-ups from others.

- If you eat dessert as part of your meal, eat less carbohydrate (starch, fruit, milk) in the rest of the meal, or learn to adjust your short or fast-acting insulin for larger portions.

When you are the host

When you are entertaining, whether it's a special family event, a religious festival or simply a get-together with friends, you have to put yourself first. Here are some tips:

- Only buy and prepare as much food as you need
- Let your guests know that there's no need to bring any food: if it is a tradition that everyone contributes something, specify exactly what you would like them to bring, and
- Freeze leftovers as soon as possible—this means you're less likely to pick at them while you are cleaning up. Better still, give leftovers to guests when they leave or donate them to a charity that feeds underprivileged or homeless people.

Christmas

Christmas is one day of the year. Try to keep your celebratory eating separate from your regular meals instead of letting the whole Christmas period become a time of gorging and indulgence. At the same time, however, don't expect to lose weight; that would just be setting yourself up for failure.

The main course: the traditional meal—whether it's roast turkey or whole fish cooked on the grill—should be OK, but you may need to keep an eye on the timing of the meal.

Dessert options: prepare or buy lots of fruit salad. There's nothing more refreshing, and it makes a wonderful light alternative to traditional Christmas desserts.

Christmas cake: take care with Christmas cake too, even if your great aunt makes one with no added sugar. Fruit cake is a very concentrated source of carbohydrate and (depending on the recipe) saturated fat, so one thick finger-sized piece would be enough at one sitting.

Because you're likely to be on vacation over the Christmas holiday, you may have time to fit in more activity. An after-meal walk or backyard game will help you digest your food and counteract the calories. Try these ideas:

- A day out at the park, zoo or indoor game center
- An adventure vacation (instead of the usual few lazy days poolside/fireside), and
- Asking for an active present, such as a gym membership, rock-climbing course, exercise machine or weekend at a health retreat.

Let people know if you don't want food—especially chocolates and sweets—as gifts.

Easter

Again, because it comes but once a year, Easter is another time when a little indulgence is OK and shouldn't upset your diabetes management too much (depending on how much you like chocolate).

Obviously you need to try to keep to regular meals, but that is usually more difficult when you're socializing or traveling, so consider taking supplies with you. A bit of fresh fruit, a sandwich—something simple that may not be easily available when you're out.

It will also help to keep your carbohydrate intake under control if you know how to substitute Easter foods for your usual carbohydrate. If the information isn't available on a food label, here are a few basics:

- Hot cross buns—work on them being about 50 percent carbohydrate, so an average bun of 80g will give you around 40g of carbohydrate.
- Jelly beans—about 14 beans totals 150 calories, 37g of carbohydrate and 27g of sugars

- Easter eggs—look for the weight and work on 100g of chocolate containing 60g (4 exchanges—see Chapter 9) of carbohydrate.
- Chocolate—the carbohydrate content varies depending on the quality of the chocolate. Most chocolate is around 50–60 percent carbohydrate. The healthiest choice is the very dark (85 percent cocoa) variety because it's richest in antioxidants and is a low 20 percent carbohydrate.

Easter eggs, being hollow, look like more chocolate than they actually are, so they aren't bad value for a child with diabetes. Easter-themed gifts could be a welcome addition to a big single chocolate egg for a child; an adult may prefer a bunch of flowers, a basket of fruit or a bottle of wine.

Don't bother with diabetic chocolate or eggs. They cost more and are still high in saturated fat and calories. They may be sugar free, but that isn't really the issue with chocolate.

The real deal on chocolate

Most people with diabetes or prediabetes can enjoy an occasional chocolate if eaten in moderation—there is increasing scientific evidence that a little bit of chocolate each day may do you good.

Chocolate and your blood glucose

Although most chocolates have a relatively high sugar content, they don't have a big impact on your blood glucose levels. In fact the average GI is around 45 because their high fat content slows the rate at which the sugars from the stomach are released into the intestine and absorbed into the blood. So people with diabetes don't need to eat low- or reduced-sugar chocolates to avoid high blood glucose levels. However, alternatively sweetened chocolates usually do have fewer calories—a big advantage if you are trying to lose weight.

Chocolate and your weight

Most chocolates are what we call energy dense—you get a lot of calories in a little piece. This is good if you are trying to gain weight, travel long distances with limited storage space, or participate in an endurance sport where it is an advantage to be able to carry around a concentrated and highly palatable source of carbohydrate and energy. But it is obviously not good if you are trying to lose weight.

If you are overweight, only buy your favorite, high quality chocolate, and take care not to eat too much. Keep it for a treat.

Chocolate and your blood fats

Chocolate is high in total and saturated fats. In high quality chocolates, cocoa butter is the main source of fat. This is important because cocoa butter is high in a particular kind of saturated fat called stearic acid. Stearic acid raises the bad LDL cholesterol less than all other saturated fats do, and it raises the good HDL cholesterol more, so the net effect on your total blood cholesterol levels is not bad at all.

However, the amount of cocoa butter—and therefore the amount of stearic acid as well—used in chocolate varies, and this information is usually not provided in any simple form on the wrapper. As a rough guide, the better quality (and therefore more expensive) varieties generally have more cocoa butter, so they are usually a better choice.

Chocolate and antioxidants

Chocolate is one of nature's richest sources of a powerful group of antioxidants known as flavonoids—others are green and black tea, red wine, certain fruits (berries, black grapes, plums, apples) and vegetables (artichokes, asparagus, cabbage, russet and sweet potatoes). It's believed that these antioxidants may benefit people with diabetes or prediabetes by helping to stop cholesterol sticking to the walls of blood vessels, relaxing major blood vessels and thereby decreasing blood pressure, and maybe even reducing the ability of the blood to form too many clots. A 1 oz piece of dark chocolate (about one row of a block) provides about the same amount of these antioxidants as half a cup of black tea or a glass of red wine.

Milk chocolate has only a third of the antioxidant dark chocolate has, and white chocolate has none at all.

Ramadan

With type 2 diabetes, there is obviously less risk of hypoglycemia during fasting, but if you overindulge at sunset and before dawn, you run a real risk of hyperglycemia. It would be better to distribute your food over three smaller meals to prevent this. It's best to make your decision about fasting after talking with your GP/diabetes team.

If you are considering fasting, see if you can have a checkup with your GP/diabetes team 1–2 months before Ramadan. Make sure you're clear about dosing and timing of medications, how often to monitor, meal planning and what to do about physical activity.

The pre-dawn meal: during Ramadan the pre-dawn meal would ideally be based on low GI carbohydrate to help sustain you throughout the day.

The evening meal: the meal at sunset may be higher GI, but it's not a good idea to follow the common practice of eating large amounts of high carbohydrate, high fat foods at this time.

Make a deliberate effort to increase your fluid intake during non-fasting times.

You will have to end the fast immediately if your blood glucose level:

- Drops below 60 mg/dL, or
- Is less than 70 mg/dL in the first few hours after starting the fast (especially if you've taken insulin or sulphonylureas pre-dawn).

Chapter 28

What to do when you get sick or go to the hospital

Managing your diabetes when you're sick is more demanding than when you're well, even though the basics don't change. You can apply the general principles we outline in this chapter to help you get through, but visit your doctor if the problem persists more than a couple of days.

First, it's important to know that some illnesses will cause your blood glucose levels to go low, and others will cause them to go high.

Infections that usually cause low blood glucose levels are generally associated with nausea, vomiting and/or diarrhea, but with no accompanying fever, and there is no increase in insulin resistance or insulin requirements. Rather, the problem seems to be mainly with your inability to absorb or retain food. Common causes are viruses associated with mild gastritis (nausea and vomiting only) or a mild gastroenteritis (vomiting and diarrhea). Food poisoning may present a similar picture.

Infections that usually cause high blood glucose levels are more common, and they are generally associated with a fever. They tend to raise blood glucose levels because they involve higher levels of stress hormones and other factors, which increase gluconeogenesis and insulin resistance. In addition, ketones may appear in the urine. Illnesses that cause raised blood glucose levels are usually those associated with feelings of lethargy, weakness, irritability, muscle aches, headache, fever and obvious signs of an infection. And remember, many of these kinds of infections have a silent phase—you may have unexplained high blood glucose levels for several days before the illness itself becomes apparent.

The essential principles in sick day management are:

- **Treat the underlying illness.** You may need to see your doctor for antibiotics or other prescription medications
- **Symptomatic relief.** If you have a fever, headache or aches and pains, take regular acetaminophen or other similar medications in recommended doses
- **Rest.** Get plenty of bed rest, and whenever possible, stay at home
- **Lower-carbohydrate medications.** For young children, many syrups are available in sugar-free forms (antibiotics, acetaminophen, ibuprofen), and those that aren't sugar free are usually OK because the amount of carbohydrate in each dose is not large enough to cause a problem. For older children, adolescents and adults, most medications are available in tablet or capsule form, and these are sugar free, and
- **Drink plenty of fluids.** People with diabetes and a fever lose fluid due to the increased body temperature; they may also be losing quite large volumes of fluid because of high blood glucose levels, which increase urination. If blood glucose levels are greater than 270 mg/dL, drink some water or low calorie drinks to avoid raising blood glucose higher.

What should be in your first-aid kit?

Everyone with diabetes should have a first aid kit prepared and ready to use when required. It should have in it:

- Local doctor's and hospital's phone number
- Journal, for recording and dating symptoms and blood glucose levels
- Thermometer
- Acetominophen or alternative
- Low calorie (diet drinks) or water
- Fruit juice/lemonade or other soft drinks (caffeine is not recommended)
- Rapid or short-acting insulin and ketone test strips (if you use insulin), and
- Glucagon (people with type 1).

What you should eat or drink when you aren't feeling well

The following drinks and foods will give you about 15g of carbohydrate and are usually well tolerated.

Beverage/food	Amount/volume
Milk	1 cup (250ml)
Milk + flavoring	¾ cup (200ml) milk + 1 tbsp Quik
Fruit juice	½–¾ cup (125–200ml)
Tea or coffee, hot water with lemon juice	Add 1 tbsp sugar or honey
Sports (electrolyte) drink	1 cup (250ml)
Pedialyte	2 packets

Beverage/food	Amount/volume
Ordinary soft drink (not low calorie or diet)	¾ cup (200ml)
Canned soup	1 cup (250ml) reconstituted
Breakfast cereals	½ cup oatmeal
Dry toast	1 slice
Crackers or crisp bread	2 Ryvita
Mashed potato	½ cup
Rice	⅓ cup
Ordinary gelatin or pudding	½ cup
Low-fat ice cream	1–1½ scoops
Popsicle	1 average

At the hospital

Generally, hospital admission is disruptive to glycemic management and to your diet—as much because it is different from your usual regimen as because of anything else. Lying in bed, invasive procedures, stress and pain, changes to medications can all increase your blood glucose levels. But good blood glucose levels are necessary for a speedy recovery, so it's important to do all you can to help keep your blood glucose in a healthy range.

A stay in the hospital is not a time to forget about your diet.

Hospital meals are very unlikely to be the same as what you eat at home. Although the food service differs from hospital to hospital, most have standard menus for people with diabetes—for meals and snacks. These days, you usually get to choose from the menu, but sometimes it can be a while before it finds you, so your first few meals are likely to have been chosen for you.

You may automatically receive a diabetic menu or you may be able to choose from the full menu. In either case, you may find limits applied to control the amount of carbohydrate you receive and to keep the meal low in saturated fat and sodium.

Sometimes you'll find you've been on the full menu by mistake, so don't assume that everything you're being offered is OK for you. If you think what you're being offered is not appropriate, say something to nursing or food service staff.

Keep in mind that hospital food service is trying to please the majority. This is why hospital food tends to be bland, soft and easy to chew. So if you need something different, ask for it. If you're finding it difficult to eat anything, for example, a restricted menu won't suit you and you'll need to ask for something else. If you usually have a snack in the evening before you go to bed and you're not receiving one, ask for it. If you are away from the ward during meal time and no food is offered to you when you return, speak up.

The general rule is talk to the dietitian, diet technician aid, nurse or doctor if things are not working.

Never assume that the nurses know you have missed your meal and that you need something.

Fluids only

You might be put on fluids only after surgery or as part of the preparation for a procedure. There are basically only two menus—free fluids or clear fluids. A clear fluid diet consists of water, juices, gelatin, lemonade, popsicles, clear soup (stock), black tea and coffee; a free fluid diet includes milk, creamy soups, mousses and ice cream. Some of the fluids will be sugar sweetened and will act as an alternative source of carbohydrate while you're not eating.

Fasting

There may be times during a hospital stay when you will be put on "fasting." This is to keep your stomach empty—before surgery, for example. Even water isn't allowed. At these times your blood glucose levels should be closely monitored, and adjustments may have to be made to your diabetes medication or insulin to control them.

Chapter 29
Do you need to take a supplement?

If you're generally healthy and eat a wide variety of foods as part of a well-balanced diet, including fruits, vegetables, dairy, whole grains, legumes and lean meats and fish, it's very unlikely that you need to take a supplement. There are some times, however, when your doctor or dietitian may recommend you take one.

If you're pregnant or planning to have a baby, a folate supplement is recommended. It helps protect your baby against neural tube birth defects such as spina bifida. As we say in Chapter 31, it's important to start taking this before you become pregnant.

Men and women over 50 may need a calcium and vitamin D supplement. This helps keep your bones strong and decrease bone loss after menopause if you don't get enough calcium and vitamin D from your diet.

Some vegetarians and vegans may need supplements. Although it is possible to meet your nutrient requirements from non-meat sources, if your diet isn't optimal, or you're going through a time of increased requirements, you may not get quite enough. Vitamin B12 is the one that can cause problems, especially for vegans, as it isn't naturally found in plant foods. So if you don't eat meat, dairy foods or eggs, your only reliable source of B12 will be fortified vegetarian foods or a dietary supplement.

When you are first diagnosed with diabetes, your blood glucose levels may have been high for some time, which means you may be deficient in a number of vitamins and minerals because many are either lost in the urine, or because the amount you need is higher because of the diabetes itself. The most common problems are the vitamins E, B6, folate, B12, and the minerals calcium, zinc, magnesium and possibly chromium. Sometimes people taking the tablet metformin develop a B12 deficiency, so a B12 supplement may be necessary.

After a few months, when your blood glucose levels have returned to normal (or close to it) through healthy eating, regular physical activity and appropriate medication, your vitamin and mineral requirements will return to normal too.

Whatever your situation is, it's best to discuss which vitamin and mineral supplements you need, if any, with your dietitian or doctor. Most of the rest of us don't need to worry about supplementation—it's just not necessary.

How common are vitamin and mineral deficiencies?

True vitamin and mineral deficiencies can result in poor wound healing, bruising, anemia, increased risk of infections, cognitive (mental) impairment, neurological disorders, stroke and some cancers. Luckily, these levels of deficiency are rare. They are usually only seen in cases of extreme poverty, or if you:

- Have a very poor diet
- Are on a very restricted weight loss diet (less than 1,200 calories a day)
- Have a medical condition such as undiagnosed celiac disease that affects how your body absorbs, uses or excretes nutrients

- Smoke—tobacco decreases the absorption of many vitamins and minerals, including vitamin C, folate, magnesium and calcium, and/or
- Drink excessively—long-term excessive alcohol consumption can impair the digestion and absorption of several vitamins and minerals, including vitamin B1, iron, zinc, magnesium and folate.

True vitamin or mineral deficiency is rare in people with diabetes. However, high blood glucose levels can lead to increased urination, which means you can lose some B group vitamins, vitamin C, and certain minerals in your urine.

On the other hand, some minerals—copper and iron, for instance—seem to be more easily stored in the bodies of people with diabetes, so taking supplements of these can be dangerous.

What's the best way to make sure you are getting enough vitamins and minerals?

The best way to ensure you are getting the right amount of all vitamins and minerals is to eat a well-balanced diet. As a rule, vitamins and minerals are absorbed more effectively from foods than they are from supplements. Also, they are usually cheaper that way—and definitely much tastier!

It can be dangerous to self-treat a vitamin or mineral deficiency without knowing the underlying cause. For example, what looks like a simple iron deficiency can be caused by internal bleeding due to a cancer somewhere in the digestive tract—this happens much too often with adults. Make sure you check out any suspected deficiency with your doctor.

Should you take a supplement "just in case"?

If you eat a healthy diet and your diabetes is well managed, but you still want some "just in case" nutrition insurance, what should you do?

Ask yourself these two questions:

- Are your blood glucose levels kept within the recommended range most of the time? If they're not, talk to your dietitian and/or diabetes educator about how you can improve your blood glucose, and
- Do you think you have clear symptoms of deficiency? If you do, see your doctor because they know your medical history best.

If you do have a vitamin or mineral deficiency, talk to your dietitian about how you can change your diet so that you get all the nutrients you need from food. Don't head straight off to the pharmacy for pills to pop.

Does it really matter if you take a supplement even if your diet isn't deficient?

Yes it does. Some vitamins and minerals can be toxic if you take them in amounts that are much more than the recommended daily allowance.

On top of this, too much of one can actually cause a deficiency of another. For example, large doses of vitamin C can decrease your body's ability to absorb vitamin B12, and large doses of zinc can interfere with the absorption of copper. So remember, no megadoses.

The chromium question

Chromium is an essential mineral. Originally, scientists thought it formed a part of a glucose tolerance factor, in combination with some B group vitamins and amino acids. However, glucose tolerance factor has never been isolated in humans or animals, or synthesized in a laboratory. No one has yet proven that it actually exists!

New research suggests that rather than being a part of the glucose tolerance factor, chromium is at the center of a very small protein molecule that helps activate insulin receptors in your body's cells. If this is true, it means that chromium may help insulin work more effectively in the cells of your body. This in turn helps your body manage blood glucose levels more effectively.

How much do you need?

A minute amount. It has been estimated that 25 micrograms a day for women and 35 micrograms a day for men is all you need. This amount is easy to get from the food you eat. Good sources are:

- Bran-based breakfast cereals and wholegrain breads and cereals
- Egg yolk
- Brewers' yeast and yeast extract
- Cheese
- Fruits such as apples, oranges and pineapples
- Vegetables such as broccoli, mushrooms, potatoes with their skin on, tomatoes
- Liver, kidney and lean meat
- Peanuts
- Oysters, and
- Some spices (pepper, chili).

What happens if you don't get enough chromium?

In the past, hospitalized patients living on intravenous nutrient solutions that lacked chromium were seen to develop high blood glucose levels. When chromium was added to the intravenous solutions, the symptoms were reversed. This sparked speculation that poor chromium intake could contribute to the development of type 2 diabetes.

Many scientists believe that people with a poor or inadequate chromium intake may be more responsive to supplementation than those who are well nourished. In other words, if your diet is low in chromium, a supplement may improve glucose control.

How do you know if you are low in chromium?

People's chromium status seems to be hard to measure. Blood, urine, nail and even hair samples have been used, but none of these seems to be ideal. Despite years of research, there is still no universally accepted way of working out whether or not a person is deficient in chromium.

Should you take a chromium supplement "just in case"?

Probably not. There are risks in taking large amounts of chromium as it accumulates in the body. What we do know is that eating a varied, balanced diet will give you all the chromium you need—remember, it's a minute amount.

Chromium studies

A number of studies have been done to see whether or not people with diabetes benefit from a chromium supplement. One study in China, showed a significant improvement in blood glucose levels after taking either 200 or 1,000 micrograms of chromium (picolinate) each day for 4 months. Other studies have shown no benefit from supplementation.

Chapter 30
What about herbal therapies?

If you check out an herbal remedies encyclopedia, you'll find hundreds of plants that have a reputation for lowering blood glucose and were once "used for treating diabetes." However, most have not been scientifically evaluated, and many are consumed regularly as part of a normal healthy diet, for example:

Herbs and spices	Vegetables	Fruit
Agrimony	Cabbage	Apples
Burdock	Celery	Blackberries
Chili pepper	Garlic	Elderberries
Coriander	Haricot beans	Guavas
Dandelion	Leeks	Hops
Ginger	Lettuce	Lemons
Juniper	Mushrooms	Limes
Licorice	Onions	Lychees
Nettles	Peas	Papayas
Sage	Potatoes	Raspberries
Tarragon	Sweet corn	
Thyme	Turnips	

How do they work?

For most of these plants very little is known about how they might work to lower blood glucose. Some of the active components that have been analyzed include:

- *Alkaloids*, which are found in mulberry, fenugreek, and black beans. They also may work by slowing the rate of digestion and absorption of carbohydrates, and possibly by reducing glucose production from the liver

- *Flavonoids*, which are found in grapes and wine, tea, cocoa and soybeans, and the herb false teak. They may help stimulate insulin release from the pancreas

- *Glucosides*, which are found in bilberry, blackberry and raspberry. They may improve insulin action in the muscles and some organs, making the insulin you produce or inject work more effectively, and

- *Propionic acid*, which is found in unripe fruits, and more specifically, the Jamaican ackee apple. It may reduce glucose stores in the liver and glucose production by the liver.

Should you use herbal remedies?

There is some evidence that some plants can decrease glucose absorption, decrease glucose production, increase insulin secretion, or improve insulin action. However, there is no evidence that plants can be a substitute for insulin, so **do not** stop taking your insulin.

However, they may be useful for people with type 2 diabetes, or those trying to prevent it, but there are issues with toxicity, potency, and quality control. Why?

A couple of reasons. First, as well as the active ingredients that may help lower blood glucose levels, herbs may contain other substances that are poisonous.

Second, the amount of the active ingredient may vary considerably from batch to batch, depending on the season, where the plant was grown and how it was processed and stored. This variation could contribute to major swings in your blood glucose levels, which may be life-threatening.

What's the solution? Herbs are probably best used as a basis for research into new medicines. When the active ingredient has been identified, it can be produced in large quantities in a purified form so that there are no accompanying toxins, the dose is always the same, and the quality is strictly controlled—basically, so you know you'll get what you are paying for. For example guanidine, from the plant goats' rue (*Galega officinalis*), provided the design template for metformin (diabex, diaformin, glucophage, etc.).

What about cinnamon?

A recent study found that by taking 1–6g of cinnamon each day for 40 days, people with type 2 diabetes experienced significant improvements in blood glucose levels, LDL cholesterol and triglycerides.

However, the researchers did not state whether or not the people in the study made any changes to their diets or physical activity levels, and as we know, eating a healthy diet and increasing physical activity levels can also improve blood glucose, cholesterol and triglyceride levels. Therefore, more research is needed to work out whether or not cinnamon itself can really help people with diabetes.

Buyer beware!

Stevia rebaudiana

Stevia is a South American herb, first discovered by scientists in the late 1800s. Its extract, stevioside, is 250–300 times sweeter than sucrose, but unlike sugars, it does not have any calories. Advertising material claims that stevia:

- "Is better . . . than pharmaceutical sweeteners"
- "May actually lower blood sugar levels," and
- "Stimulates mental alertness, counters fatigue, facilitates digestion, regulates metabolism, and has a therapeutic effect on the liver, pancreas and spleen."

Despite all the claims, there has been very little scientific research done on the therapeutic properties of stevia, and what has been done suggests that it is little more than a non-nutritive alternative sweetener (see Chapter 15).

Tahitian noni juice

Noni (*Morinda citrifolia*) is a shrub or small tree that is native to Southeast Asia but has spread extensively throughout India, and into the Pacific Islands as far as Tahiti. The fruit has a pungent odor when ripening and is therefore also known as cheese fruit or even vomit fruit. Tahitian noni juice is extracted from the fruit and mixed with large quantities of "natural fruit juices" (such as blackcurrant), then sold as a tonic—noni juice. It is supposed to contain the active ingredient "xeronine," which is claimed to:

- Lower blood pressure
- Regulate sleep, temperature and moods
- Increase body energy
- Alleviate pain
- Have antibacterial properties, and
- Inhibit growth of cancer tumors and autoimmune diseases.

Unfortunately, there is no evidence so far that Tahitian noni juice has any therapeutic benefits for humans, so it seems to be little more than a very expensive fruit juice!

PREGNANCY, BIRTH, BREASTFEEDING AND DIABETES

A woman with diabetes has just as much chance of having a healthy baby as anyone else these days, if her diabetes is well controlled before and during pregnancy and her general health is good. So, if you have diabetes, want to have a baby and are trying to make it happen, make sure you're in as good health as you can be. If you don't want to get pregnant, take precautions to make sure it doesn't happen. Unplanned pregnancy with poorly managed diabetes can cause a lot of heartbreak to all involved.

Chapter 31

Diabetes during pregnancy, birth and while breastfeeding

In this chapter we cover some of the steps you need to take as you prepare for pregnancy. We focus on the nutritional needs of pregnancy for you and your baby, and on how you can best meet these while managing your diabetes and controlling your blood glucose. We also give you the answers to the questions we are most often asked about pregnancy and diabetes.

Planning for pregnancy

Your blood glucose levels need to be as good as you can possibly get them *before you conceive*. This is because the first eight weeks (often before you know you are pregnant) is a critical time for your baby's development. It is when the major organs are formed, and optimal blood glucose management is vital. So make some appointments before you start trying for a baby.

**Optimal diabetes management for pregnancy means
HbA1c less than 1 percent above the reference range
(generally less than 7 percent or 53 mmol/mol).**

Who you should see before you get pregnant

Your doctor or diabetes specialist: to discuss what you can do to improve your blood glucose levels and whether any of your medications will need to be changed.

If you have type 2 diabetes and you take pills to manage your blood glucose levels, your doctor or diabetes specialist will usually advise you to use insulin from early pregnancy. They will also check your vitamin B12 levels if you've been taking metformin.

Talk to your doctor about any other medications you take as well, including blood pressure and cholesterol medications. Sometimes you have to change medications or stop taking some while you're pregnant.

Some diabetic complications, such as retinopathy and nephropathy, can be made worse by pregnancy. Your doctor will want you to have an eye check (including examination of the retina). If you need laser therapy, do it before you get pregnant. Your kidneys will need to be checked too, and your doctor will also check for major blood vessel disease. In some cases, sadly, the doctor may even advise against trying for a baby.

Your diabetes educator and dietitian: to discuss your diet and exercise program and make sure you know how to deal with morning sickness, hypoglycemia and sick days.

As you already know, a major part of good diabetes management is eating healthily. If you begin your pregnancy well nourished, what you eat during pregnancy is not so critical. However, if you've been eating poorly before you get pregnant, a healthy diet during pregnancy is very important to the health of your baby.

You'll also be advised to take 5 mg of folic acid (folate) a day, from at least one month before conception and throughout the first three months, to help prevent neural tube defects.

> ### Stop!
>
> If you smoke, quit before conception. Smoking harms the development of your baby.
>
> If you drink, give it up. Alcohol increases the risk of miscarriage and birth defects.
>
> If you use recreational drugs, stop. Like alcohol, these substances increase the risk of miscarriage and birth defects.

You and your team

Managing your diabetes well during your pregnancy means working with a team of health professionals, which may include:

- Diabetes specialist/endocrinologist
- Dietitian
- Obstetrician
- Midwife, and
- Diabetes educator.

Diabetes and pregnancy clinics at large hospitals generally have all these professionals.

Your diet during pregnancy

There are some wonderful changes that occur in your body during pregnancy (and some not so wonderful) to create the most favorable environment for the development of your baby. One of these changes relates to how your body absorbs nutrients. The recommended daily intakes (RDI) for almost all nutrients are increased in pregnancy, and it is clear that your absorption of nutrients increases noticeably when you're pregnant (and breastfeeding) to meet these demands. This in part is thanks to progesterone, a hormone secreted by the placenta: it slows down your digestive tract, giving more time for nutrient absorption. (Incidentally, the slowing down of the digestive tract also contributes to constipation—that's the not so wonderful part.)

The key to providing these important nutrients is the food you eat. As long as you have had a nutritious diet before pregnancy and continue with it during pregnancy, you should be able to meet the recommended nutrient needs without a supplement. There are two possible exceptions—folate and iron.

To help ensure your diet gives you all the nutrients you need, these are some general guidelines:

- Eat as wide a variety of nutritious foods as possible
- Limit fatty foods, especially those high in saturated fat
- Limit foods and drinks containing large amounts of refined or added sugar or starch with low nutritive value such as soft drinks, candy, chips and other packaged snacks, and
- Avoid alcohol.

Coping with morning sickness

The biggest influence on your diet when you are first pregnant is probably whether or not you get morning sickness—and if you do, how badly. "Morning" is a bit of a misnomer, as it can happen any time of day (or even last all day). Being tired seems to make it worse. Symptoms can range from periodic mild nausea to constant nausea and vomiting (such as hyperemesis).

Unfortunately, no one has yet come up with the ideal solution as to what's best to eat to help morning sickness. The ideas on the following page may be useful:

- Aim to eat small amounts of carbohydrate-based foods or drinks frequently over the day. An empty stomach can make you feel worse.
- Keep your fluids up, particularly if you're vomiting. If you are unable to eat and your blood glucose levels are less than 270 mg/dL, sip on flat lemonade, fruit juice or popsicles. If your blood glucose level is greater than 15 mmol/l, sip on low calorie fluids. If plain water makes you throw up, try crushed ice.
- If mornings are a problem, try something first thing, before getting out of bed, such as plain water crackers or dry toast. A box of crackers by the bed can be handy.
- Salty foods are sometimes better tolerated, so nibble guiltlessly on pretzels, potato chips or salty crackers if they are the only food that stays down.
- Fatty foods make some women feel worse, but for others it's what they feel like, so try different things and see what suits you best.
- Ginger has anti-nausea properties, so ginger tea, ale or chews can be helpful.
- You'll probably be aware that smells can really set some women off, so let those around you know if you want to avoid perfumes, bad breath or the smell of certain foods.

Managing your blood glucose levels

This can present quite a challenge—to you, and to your diabetes team. We don't really know exactly why pregnancy affects blood glucose levels so powerfully, but one cause is a hormone called placental lactogen, which increases insulin resistance by up to 50 percent. This makes it more difficult for the mother's body to take up glucose, which means higher blood glucose levels.

The most important part of your diet to monitor is carbohydrates because they have the greatest effect on your blood glucose. You need to be clear about which foods are sources of carbohydrate and how they affect your blood glucose levels. You also need to know the low GI foods that can help you manage your blood glucose levels better. If you take insulin, make sure you know how your insulin dose relates to the amount of carbohydrate you eat and how long your insulin lasts—you may need more snacks.

Home blood glucose monitoring will give you invaluable information on the impact of food on your blood glucose levels—we encourage all women whose pregnancy is complicated by diabetes to do this. Recommended testing times will vary, but many women test four times a day, including in the morning after an overnight fast and two hours after main meals. If you are using insulin, it's a good idea to test before meals as well. Make sure you check the results of your monitoring with a health professional regularly. Together you can plan adjustments to your insulin (if you take it) and diet to improve your blood glucose levels.

Your baby and blood glucose

Glucose crosses freely from your blood into the baby through the placenta. Your baby makes its own insulin from about 15 weeks, to handle this glucose. If your blood glucose level is high, higher levels of glucose will be transferred to your baby. This stimulates your baby's pancreas to make extra insulin. The extra insulin makes your baby grow bigger and fatter than normal, which presents complications for labor and delivery. It is also believed to have an adverse effect on the baby's later health—obesity and diabetes are more common in children born to women with diabetes.

Q&A

When I have low blood sugar, does my baby have it too?

No. When your blood glucose is low, it doesn't affect your baby the way it affects you. Babies can maintain their blood glucose by releasing glucose from their liver if there isn't enough glucose coming through the placenta.

Does the insulin I take affect my baby?

Insulin that you take by injection or pump, or insulin that your own body produces, does not cross the placenta. However, insulin that you take has an indirect effect on your baby because of its effect on your blood glucose levels. That's why it's so important to manage your blood glucose levels with insulin really carefully.

If your blood glucose levels go too high, your baby may grow bigger and fatter than normal, and the risk of developing a range of birth defects increases. If they go too low, you and your baby are at risk of accidents, injury, even unconsciousness or death.

Will my baby be born with diabetes?

No. However, if your blood glucose levels are not managed well during pregnancy, your baby may be at increased risk of becoming overweight and obese and developing type 2 diabetes later in life.

What to expect after delivery

Your blood glucose levels will fall after delivery, and if you took insulin during your pregnancy, you may not need it now. You may well be able to keep your blood glucose levels down just through your diet, especially if you are breastfeeding. If you need medication to manage your blood glucose levels, insulin is recommended—pills are OK, but be aware that some, such as metformin, can be passed through to your baby through breast milk.

Breastfeeding

Your blood glucose levels may fall rapidly during and after breastfeeding.

A blood glucose test before feeding will give you an indication of whether or not your insulin dose is correct—and an idea of how much carbohydrate you might need for a snack. It's important to get it right: not enough insulin may inhibit milk production, and too much causes low blood sugar, which stimulates the release of adrenaline, which in turn inhibits milk production.

> **If my blood sugar is high, will my breast milk be higher in sugar too?**
>
> No. Your blood glucose concentration does not affect the glucose concentration of your breast milk.

Don't worry if you feel hungry all the time. Like all new mothers, you do need to eat more when you are breastfeeding: 475 calories per day extra is recommended. For a typical woman, this means eating about 25 percent more food than usual. You'll probably find that your appetite will increase. Your carbohydrate requirements may vary according to your baby's feeding pattern. When your baby is feeding a lot, you may need to increase your carbohydrates; and maybe you'll need to cut down if your baby is unwell or if she/he is feeding less.

Diet tips while breastfeeding

- Snack before or while feeding: keep a glass of milk or fruit juice handy
- Drink at least 68 ounces of fluids a day, and
- Test your blood glucose levels after you feed your baby, especially during the night, to prevent nocturnal hypoglycemia, and consider a reduction in long-acting insulin if nocturnal hypoglycemia does occur.

Chapter 32
Diabetes during pregnancy and breastfeeding: Your daily food guides

During pregnancy there is a small increase in energy requirements during the second and third trimesters of pregnancy, but you don't have to eat for two. Only about 300 calories per day extra are required—two extra servings of fruit plus an extra meat or vegetarian serving, for example. It is important that the extra calories come from nutrient-rich foods. If you are eating the suggested minimum daily servings of each food group, your appetite is your best guide to whether you are eating enough, unless you are gaining too much weight.

Your daily food guide during pregnancy

- 6–10 servings breads, cereals and other starchy foods
- 2–3 servings fruits
- 2 servings milk products
- 3 servings meat or vegetarian alternatives
- 3 servings fat-rich foods, and
- 5–6 servings vegetables.

The daily food guide provides between 1,800–2,250 calories, with 40 to 50 percent of energy from carbohydrate. At the lower calorie level, iron (15 mg) and folate (500 mcg) contents are less than the recommended daily intake (RDI) for pregnancy (27 mg and 600 mcg, respectively), so a supplement is recommended. At the higher calorie level, the iron content meets the average requirement, but a supplement would still be a good idea if you are not eating iron-fortified foods. Serving sizes can be found on pages 152 and 153.

How do you fit this into a day?

This sample meal plan illustrates one way of distributing the recommended servings of foods over the day. For a meal plan that is individualized to your needs, we suggest you consult a dietitian.

Meal plan for pregnancy	Daily food servings	Example	Other ideas
Breakfast	2 servings bread, cereal or other starchy food	¾ cup Special K (original) with ½ cup All-Bran	toast, muesli, oatmeal or a low GI cereal
	1 serving milk product	1 cup lower fat milk	milk or yogurt for cereal
Snack	2 servings bread, cereal or other starchy food with 1 serving fat-rich food	2 slices grain toast topped with 2 tsp canola spread	wholegrain crackers with avocado

Meal plan for pregnancy	Daily food servings	Example	Other ideas
Lunch	2 servings bread, cereal or other starchy food + 1 serving fat	2 fresh medium corn cobs with 1 tsp margarine	2 thick slices of wholegrain bread
	1 serving fruit	⅓ canteloupe	diced apple
	1 serving meat or alternative	100g can tuna	60g cheddar cheese
	2 servings vegetables + 1 serving fat	2 cups chopped mixed salad vegetables with 1 tbsp dressing	lettuce, celery, walnuts and mayonnaise
Snack	1 serving vegetables + 1 serving fruit	1 large glass fresh squeezed carrot and apple juice	commercial fruit and vegetable juice boxes
Dinner	2 servings bread, cereal or other starchy food	1 cup hokkien noodles	rice, chickpeas
	2 servings meat or alternative	200g lean beef strips	chicken, fish
	3 servings vegetables + ½ serving fat-rich food	stir-fried mix of broccoli, onion, bell pepper, snow peas, baby corn	at least 1½ cups cooked vegetables
Snack/dessert	1 serving milk product	1 cup lower fat fruit yogurt	milk, low-fat ice cream
	1 serving fruit	½ cup diced peach and pear	any fresh, dried or canned fruit

What if I'm breastfeeding?

During lactation you need to eat more from most food groups, except meat and alternatives because your iron needs are not as high as they are during pregnancy. An average* guide should include the following:

- 8–10 servings breads, cereals and other starchy foods
- 4–5 servings fruits
- 2 servings milk products
- 2 servings meat or vegetarian alternatives
- 3 servings fat-rich foods, and
- 6+ servings vegetables.

*The daily food guide provides 1,975–2,200 calories, with 50 percent of energy coming from carbohydrate. It meets the RDI for all the nutrients for which we have food composition data.

How do you fit this into a day?

It might look like a lot of food—let your appetite guide you with quantities if you are in doubt.

Meal plan for breastfeeding	Daily food servings	Example
Breakfast	4 servings bread, cereals or other starchy foods	2 slices thick-cut wholegrain bread
	1 serving vegetables	pan-fried tomato, spinach, mushroom and onion
	1 serving meat or alternative	2 omega-3 rich eggs
	1 serving fruit	a small apple juice
Snack	1 serving fruit with 2 servings fat-rich foods	60g mixed dried fruit and nuts

Meal plan for breastfeeding	Daily food servings	Example
Lunch	3 servings bread, cereal or other starchy foods	one round of flatbread
	½ serving meat or alternative	a couple of thin slices of cooked chicken or beef
	3 servings vegetables	tomato, onion, lettuce
	1 serving milk product	a glass of low-fat milk
Snack	1 serving milk product with 1 serving fruit	1 cup of mixed berries with 1 cup of vanilla yogurt
Dinner	½ serving meat or alternative	30g grated parmesan cheese
	2 servings other starchy foods	1 cup of cooked pasta
	3 servings vegetables	1½ cups tomato and vegetable pasta sauce
	1 serving fruit	handful of black grapes
Snack/dessert	1 serving bread or cereal 1 serving fat-rich food	a slice of raisin toast topped with margarine
	1 serving fruit	a couple of fresh plums

Resources

Glycemic Index
www.glycemicindex.com
http://ginews.blogspot.com

American Diabetes Association (ADA)
800-DIABETES (800-342-2383)
www.diabetes.org

American Association of Diabetes Educators (AADE)
800-338-3633
www.aadenet.org

American Dietetic Association
800-877-1600
www.eatright.org

Canadian Diabetes Association
800-BANTING (800-226-8464)
www.diabetes.ca

Canadian Diabetes Educator Certification Board
905-838-4898
www.cdecb.ca

Dietitians of Canada
416-596-0857
www.dieticians.ca

Stop Smoking
United States: 800-QUIT-NOW (800-784-8669)
smokefree.gov

Canada: 866-225-0709
Health Canada: hc-sc.gc.ca

Index

About the authors

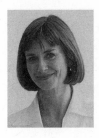

PROFESSOR JENNIE BRAND-MILLER (AM) is Professor of Human Nutrition at the Charles Perkins Centre, University of Sydney. She is recognized around the world for her work on carbohydrates and the glycemic index of foods. She received the 2003 Clunies Ross Medal for contributions to science and technology in Australia. She is a past President of the Nutrition Society of Australia, past Chair of the National Committee for Nutrition of the Australian Academy of Science, and President of the Glycemic Index Foundation Limited, a not-for-profit company that administers a food symbol for consumers in partnership with the Juvenile Diabetes Research Foundation (Australia). Jennie is the proud recipient of two Nucleus bionic ears.

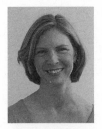

KAYE FOSTER-POWELL is an Accredited Practicing Dietitian with extensive experience in diabetes management. Currently she is senior dietitian with Nepean Blue Mountains Diabetes Service.

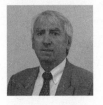

PROFESSOR STEPHEN COLAGIURI is Professor of Metabolic Health at Sydney University. He has extensive clinical and research experience in the management of diabetes and metabolic problems.

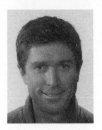

DR. ALAN BARCLAY is an Accredited Practicing Dietitian and Accredited Nutritionist and worked for Diabetes Australia from 1998 to 2014, most recently as Head of Research. He is currently the Chief Scientific Officer of the Glycemic Index Foundation.

Acknowledgments

We are indebted to our ever-cheerful, ever-encouraging publishing team at Hachette Australia, and in particular Fiona Hazard and Karen Ward.

We really appreciate the generosity of the people who shared their "success stories" with us. Our thanks also to Peter Howard and Diane Temple. To the people who work at Diabetes Australia, the Juvenile Diabetes Research Foundation and Diabetes NZ, we acknowledge the vital role you play and resources you provide to improve the lives of people with diabetes.

Many dietitians and colleagues gave us useful feedback at various stages of the publishing process, thank you one and all. In addition, Alan would like to thank Kaye, Peter, Trisha, Brian, Melanie and Michael Peters for their helpful comments. We would also like to thank the people who keep the GI database at the University of Sydney up to date: Associate Professor Gareth Denyer and Fiona Atkinson, Manager of the Sydney University Glycemic Index Research Service.

We are most grateful to our agent, Philippa Sandall, for holding on to the vision for this book and making it a reality.

Lastly, we thank our wonderful families – John Miller; Ruth Colagiuri; and Sharon, Marcus and Michael Barclay for their encouragement and support.